NN 611
E 18.50 T

72.90

Doctors Afield

DOCTORS AFIELD

EDITED BY

Mary G. McCrea Curnen

Howard Spiro

and Deborah St. James

Prepared under the auspices
of the Program for Humanities in Medicine
Yale University School of Medicine

Yale University Press   New Haven and London

Designed by Sonia L. Scanlon
Set in Adobe Garamond with Gill Sans display type by
Running Feet Books, Morrisville, North Carolina
Printed in the United States of America by Vail-Ballou Press,
Binghamton, New York

Library of Congress Cataloging-in-Publication Data
Doctors afield / edited by Mary G. McCrea Curnen,
Howard Spiro, and Deborah St. James ; prepared under the
auspices of the Program for Humanities in Medicine,
Yale University School of Medicine.
p. cm.
ISBN 0–300–08020–4 (alk. paper)
1. Physicians—United States Biography. I. Curnen,
Mary G. McCrea, 1922– . II. Spiro, Howard M.
(Howard Marget), 1924– . III. St. James,
Deborah, 1947– . IV. Yale University. Program for
Humanities in Medicine.
R134.5.D63   1999
610' .92'273—dc21   99–28479
[B]   CIP

A catalogue record for this book is available
from the British Library.

The paper in this book meets the guidelines for
permanence and durability of the
Committee on Production Guidelines for
Book Longevity of the Council on Library Resources.

10 9 8 7 6 5 4 3 2 1

In loving memory of Edward C. Curnen, Jr., M.D.,
the late husband of Mary G. McCrea Curnen, whose support
and counsel were vital to this book. Throughout his creative life,
he was truly an inspiration to doctors afield.

Mary G. McCrea Curnen
Howard Spiro
Deborah St. James

Contents

Foreword

"What is there odd about being a lawyer and being or doing something else at the same time?" remarked Wallace Stevens, a lawyer, insurance executive and, in the opinion of many, the preeminent American poet of our time. A successful career in the insurance world was not a barrier to his after-hours immersion, writing poetry. Stevens was able to summon his Muse once his insurance workday had ended. Another brilliant American poet, William Carlos Williams, combined a passion for poetry with a professional career as a family doctor. Williams, however, did not accomplish his foray afield as easily as Stevens. A passage from Williams's autobiographical novel, *A Voyage to Pagany*, describes the tension and torment that these dual interests caused the writer-doctor: "Evans [the main character] had practiced medicine all his adult life, so far, up to his present fortieth year, in a continuously surly mood at the overbearing necessity for it—wanting always to do something else: to write! Why? Because then only, when he was stealing time for his machine and paper, did he live!"

The lawyer-poet was free to embrace as his own what the doctor-poet felt he must steal. This reflects the different demands between a career in law and a career in medicine. The physician is not in control of time as he or she attends to the details of patients' lives and participates in the dilemmas they face. Even when free time exists, the emotional demands of doctoring may limit the amount of creative energy available, a necessity for writing. It would therefore not seem odd to think of physicians as one-dimensional: having a singular yet admirable focus on their patients' health. Yet the opposite is true; innumerable physicians pursue their creative needs as extensions of, or departures from, their demanding lives in medicine.

For some, like the novelist-philosopher Walker Percy, an illness may direct one's calling in a new direction. Percy's convalescence from tuberculosis allowed him to engage in a period of intense reading, sparking a philosophical quest that supplanted his original plans to be a pathologist. For many other physicians, studying and writing about medical history are natural extensions of medicine. This is an example of a harmonious blending of careers wherein an avocation is an enrichment of one's vocation. Oliver Sacks and John Berger have both used the stories of their patients' lives to better understand the wonders and sorrows of the human condition.

A less harmonious blending characterized William Carlos Williams's immersion in medicine and writing. Stealing time from his medicine was necessitated by an ineluctable passion for expressing himself through poetry. Williams was seized, as are many other physician-writers, with coming to terms with Wallace Stevens's definition of the nobility of poetry as a "violence from within that protects us from a violence without." Poetry and prose may help heal the traditional "healer" and mollify the emotional demands of doctoring.

Doctors Afield incorporates many domains. It is not surprising that surgeons might find sculpting the aesthetic counterpart to their technical dexterity in the operating room, or that religiously oriented physicians might extend their care to a spiritual dimension. The clinician's gaze may also inform and direct a photographer's lens or an artist's hands. The oenophile-physician may have chemistry as an interest, and the toy maker an enchantment for play. In the past, it has also been common for physicians to play a prominent role in the political sphere. A subtext of the Flexner report required physicians to be broadly educated to prepare them to assume leadership roles in their communities. The fields to which physicians strayed were and are natural extensions of their years spent in medicine and the skills they developed during that time.

Whatever fields may capture physicians' fancies, the phenomenon attests to the continued presence of creative energy in their lives. In spite of (or because of) the heavy demands of their professional lives, physicians' passions have not been exhausted. A sense of adventure and exploration leads doctors afield into realms that complement or supplant their calling in medicine, and we are the richer for these strayings. *Doctors Afield* splendidly documents these myriad journeys.

Thomas P. Duffy, M.D.

Preface

To practice their profession, doctors need patients, but to enjoy a craft or hobby they need only themselves—and some leisure time. Medicine has become such a consuming enterprise that a doctor's identity often becomes inseparable from his or her role as a healer. That is why retired physicians continue to answer the phone, "Hello, this is Dr. So-and-So"—for they never get out of the habit of being a doctor. But this book proves just the opposite. Some physicians take up a relaxing pastime such as golf or tennis; others find creative outlets for their passion.

A few physicians know by the time of graduation that medicine is not their calling, so they write or preach or go to law school, earning a living in some other way. Others remain entranced by their medical work and in midlife find themselves so bursting with enthusiasm about what they have learned from medical practice that they begin to write stories—usually memoirs of their patients or of themselves. Now that pathography, the account of illness from both the doctor's and the patient's viewpoints, has become so popular, more and more doctors see their stories in print, though only a fortunate few achieve esteem in their new field.

Many doctors turn to music; the number of string trios or quartets composed of physicians abound. Music, after all, was grouped with arithmetic, geometry, and astronomy among the quadrivia—those fields concerned with measurement, which medicine has always found seductive—as opposed to the more verbal trivia. Religion too has held a strong attraction for physicians over the ages, however burnished their reputation as agnostics and atheists. After all, one cannot find the soul in a dissection; a lifetime of attending patients leaves most physicians aware of mysteries they cannot explain. Medical missionaries are numerous even today. Albert Schweitzer, probably as well known for his theology and music as for his medical life in Lambaréné, Gabon, has been the inspiration for many other doctors.

Larry Mellon went to medical school late in life and then went to work in Haiti, where he built the Albert Schweitzer Hospital. At Yale, Peter Parker graduated from the divinity school and medical school in the same year (1834), with the stipulation that he not practice either calling in the United States, for reasons still uncertain. He went to Canton, beginning as a surgeon to Chinese patients, and ended up as a politician instrumental in the opening of China to the West. Of course, physicians have provided a model for philosophers, from the early days of Plato and Aristotle to the present.

Most physicians who go afield continue to practice medicine, sharing their time with their new passion. Others leave medicine behind to follow an avocation that has turned into a vocation. A few never get around to practicing medicine at all. As the reader will discover, the testimonies of these men and women point to the personal gratification and the inspiration they gained from integrating medicine with another activity. Many find that the partnership enhances their ability to care for their patients or to teach.

Until the nineteenth century, medicine was simply the way that a man got an education. (Women began to be admitted to the profession only in the early twentieth century; Yale, for example, accepted its first female medical student in 1916.) Among the first Europeans in North America, the clergy, in addition to their spiritual calling, were also likely to be adept at caring for the sick; as late as the eighteenth century it was not unusual for the intelligent English or American layperson to know as much as more formally trained practitioners, or at least to be as effective in that era when caring counted for more than curing. In America that situation came to an end with the establishment of the first medical schools: the University of Pennsylvania in 1765, the College of Physicians and Surgeons at Columbia in 1767, and Harvard Medical School in 1782.

In an enchanting modern collection entitled *The Physician as a Man of Letters, Science and Action* (Glasgow: Jackson, Wylie and Co., 1933; rpt. 1951), Thomas Monro gave short biographical accounts of 593 physicians, all men who had gone afield during their lives. His volume was a testimonial to the British Empire; 196 pages were devoted to British "medical men" and the remaining 50 to continental, American, and "other foreign" physicians. It is beguiling to dip into these pages, which remind readers that some who gained great fame in other fields are rarely thought of as the physicians they were. From John Keats and Oliver Goldsmith to Sir Thomas Browne and Sir Arthur Conan Doyle, other men of "letters, science and action" range from Saint Luke, the gospel maker, to philosophers such as John Locke; from explorers such as David Livingston to pirates such as the once well known Thomas Dover (1660–1742), who plundered the high seas as a privateer after studying medicine at Cambridge. Amusingly, he reversed the modern sequence; having become rich, Dover then had the leisure to practice medicine in Bristol and London.

Between 1952 and 1969 the *New England Journal of Medicine* carried a series of columns under the general rubric "Doctors Afield." In admiration of that rich collection, which was never put together as a book but certainly deserves to be republished, we have purloined the title for this volume. Joseph Garland, the editor of the *New England Journal* in those days, was himself a good example of a doctor who had abandoned medical practice; although he began as a practicing pediatrician (one of the editors of this collection was among his first patients), he ended up working as a writer and editor for many years.

The list of doctors afield is endless because, after all, physicians vary as much as anyone else in personality, ambition, and talent. In putting this collection together, we had no particular method. We simply thought it was a good idea. At first, we somewhat randomly contacted physicians in the environs of New Haven; gradually, however, we moved farther out. Our criteria were simple: the subject of the biography or autobiography had to have attended or graduated from medical school and had to have won some repute outside medicine. In the past few decades, New Haven has fostered a school of writers who are surgeons (Sherwin Nuland, Richard Selzer, Bernie Siegel, and others), but such luminaries have already told their stories. Here we want to document the accounts of humbler writers and artists, whose successes seemed achievable and might serve as inspiration for other physicians thinking of moving afield. We made exceptions for Carlo Levi and Gertrude Stein, in that the authors of those pieces provided us with such delightful counterparts to the other stories.

As the search continued, we surveyed contemporaries, all of whom were graduates of medical schools (except for Gertrude Stein, who attended Johns Hopkins Medical School for four years but did not graduate) and widely known for their second careers. We asked them to describe what they had obtained from their dual careers and how those second careers had helped their practice of medicine and their patients.

We have assembled twenty-seven accounts, twenty-one by men and six by women. In our search for subjects, we chose not to include any physician-lawyers, as legal medicine has become almost a specialty within our profession. Our classification of "afield activities" was largely retrospective after we had enlisted our twenty-seven subjects, a number limited by the constraints of publication. For that reason, the number of accounts in each category should not be taken to reflect the proportion of physicians in the general medical population. The eight categories are as follows: the visual arts (painting, photography, sculpture); music (performance and composition); literature; astronautics; the spiritual life; government and university; collecting (cartography and numismatics); and fun and games (enology and toy making). A few of our authors fall into several classifications, as will become evident.

Over the past few years, managed care has succeeded in eliminating waste, inefficiency, and duplication, but it has left physicians bereft of time to enhance the patient-physician relationship that has guided medical practice for centuries. Doctors frustrated by the strictures imposed on them may even be considering leaving medicine. We hope this book will inspire physicians to keep practicing but to find fulfillment in another calling as well—and to have fun in the process!

Our intent was to provide a book that would let the everyday practitioner understand that he or she has stories to tell, roads to walk, pictures to paint, tunes to play—and that there is life outside, even after, medicine.

Mary G. McCrea Curnen, M.D., Dr.P.H.
Howard Spiro, M.D.

Acknowledgments

A distinguished group of physicians has given generously of their time and talent to tell us when and why they went afield and how that journey influenced their lives. We thank them all. We are also grateful to the biographers of the four subjects who are deceased and to the writers who assisted some in composing their essays.

Over the years, our Program for Humanities in Medicine has offered a lecture series that has widened the medical horizon by bringing the treasured world of the humanities to medical students, nurses, other health-care professionals, and the public at large. For this we are indebted to Clara and Frank Gyorgyey; Myra Low; Priscilla Norton and her late husband, Will Norton; Patricia Perona; and all those who faithfully support this voluntary program.

We greatly appreciate the invaluable assistance of Diane Redding, who from beginning to end brought this book to life. We are also indebted to her associates, Christina Andriole and Jennifer Ewing, who worked unceasingly on the preparation of manuscripts, diskettes, and illustrations. Without their help, this book would never have seen the light of day.

Our gratitude goes also to Vincent Giroud and Judith A. Schiff for guiding us through the illustrations in the Beinecke Rare Book and Manuscript Library at Yale University.

We thank most sincerely Jean Thomson Black, science editor at Yale University Press; Karen Gangel, manuscript editor; and many of their colleagues who assisted us in the publication of this book.

Our contributors have generously agreed to have all proceeds from this book go to the Program for Humanities in Medicine at Yale.

Last but not least, our gratitude goes to the Bayer Corporation, Pharmaceutical Division, for supporting the publication of this book and for distributing it to physicians throughout the United States.

Part 1

The Visual Arts

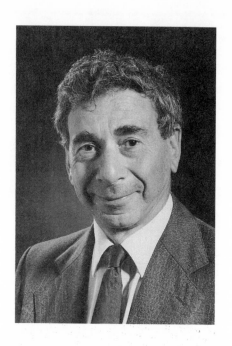

SIR ROY CALNE is a British transplant surgeon whose distinguished medical career has been coupled with an aesthetic for painting. Although his main research interest lies in immunology and graft rejection, he finds that painting or drawing his patients' portraits helps him to understand them better. Children who are allowed to color his drawings of them reveal their inner feelings in the process. Patients like to pose for Sir Roy because, as he puts it, they are "pleased at the chance of sitting, so they can talk to the surgeon about little things."

Why I Paint

Sir Roy Calne, M.D.

I decided to be a doctor, specifically, a surgeon, when I was twelve years old. I had always been fascinated by machines and how they worked, and biology gave this fascination a new dimension. Living organisms were far more exciting than engines, and even our teachers could only guess at the way some organs contributed to the well-being of the whole organism. My father was a car engineer and had served as an apprentice at the Rover car company in Coventry; it was from him I learned the hands-on enjoyment of taking mechanical things apart and putting them together again. It seemed to me that the biology of people would be more interesting to study than the mechanics of a car, and for this reason I decided on surgery at an age when my only idea about surgery involved the vaguest concepts of being an engineer for the human body.

Drawing and painting, although different from medicine and surgery, were not entirely divorced. My interest in both botany and zoology centered on structural elements, which I learned by producing anatomical drawings of plants and animals. The function of their parts did not make sense to me without a mechanistic view of their interrelationships. I often enjoyed painting landscapes, flowers, and animals from the nonanatomical point of view, and therefore from an early age I was interested in art from the point of view of both map making and aesthetic image. I received a fine background in art during secondary school, though at no time did I seriously consider painting as a profession.

When I became a medical student, the mechanistic approach to disease was again stimulated by a course in pathology, which involves the study of deviations in the structure and function of an organ; as a student I did inquire as to whether diseased kidneys could be replaced—well before such transplantations were being done. The analogy of spare parts for an engine could not have been far away in my mind, but I was told it was not possible, and in fact my tutor at medical school was not even prepared to discuss the subject. A kidney graft seemed to me to be a very simple solution to cure a young patient who was about my age and was assigned to my care. He was "kept comfortable" until he died, but I was deeply affected by that unnecessary death and sadness.

A student embarking on a career of surgery spent some time studying anatomy and teaching the subject to medical students. This I did at Oxford, where a visiting lecturer, Peter Medawar, gave a talk to the students about his work on transplanting skin. He explained how he and his colleagues had shown that skin grafts took initially but then were destroyed by a process that left a memory of the original donor, so that a second graft from the same donor would also be destroyed almost immediately. He also illustrated the most fascinating genetic experiments of a graft. During development, the immune system will accept as a "friend" foreign tissues that would otherwise be reacted against and destroyed. But when Professor Medawar was asked by a student if his studies might have therapeutic applications in the clinic, he replied with two words, "absolutely none," which I found difficult to accept in view of the positive experiments that he had described.

After qualifying as a surgeon, I was eager to learn about organ transplantation. The literature at that time was easy to read, because it was fragmentary, although scientists were trying to stop rejection by giving lethal doses of irradiation to the whole body and reconstituting the bone marrow that had been destroyed with bone marrow from the donor. That was too severe a treatment for a patient already sick with a fatal disease. I felt that some other approach would be necessary if we were going to achieve consistent success in the clinic. A report describing how antibody response to foreign protein could be prevented by the antileukemia drug 6-mercaptapurine led me to start experimenting with this compound in animals with kidney grafts, some of which had far better rates of acceptance. This success led me into further experiments and a chance to work abroad with Dr. Joseph Murray, who later won the Nobel Prize for medicine. I developed chemical immunosuppression for kidney grafting further, but the initial results were disappointing. Still, the addition of steroids made it possible to begin clinical organ transplantation with a reasonable chance of some long-term success. For twenty years we tried to find safer and more specific immunosuppression, but it was not until 1977 that cyclosporin, a fungal product, proved effective. We were dismayed to find that although this drug did not damage animal kidneys, it was nephrotoxic in humans, and we had to learn from bitter experience how to use it.

I began clinical liver transplantation in Europe in 1968. In humans, liver grafts are rejected unless immunosuppression is given. We learned how to manage immunosuppressive drugs in recipients of liver allografts and also how to do the operation with reasonable success.

All my life I had been painting, mainly as a relaxation during holidays. I had learned to use the long Chinese brush for flower painting in the Chinese style from Earl Lu, a friend and surgical colleague in Singapore. I had also taken watercolor courses with Ron Ranson in England, in the Wye Valley. So by the 1970s my interest and time spent in painting were increasing. One of my patients at that time was the distinguished Scottish painter John Bellany, who underwent a liver transplant in my department; during his three-week recuperation, he did sixty paintings of himself, filling his room and the corridors. These powerful images showed a heroic figure often suffering at the hands of doctors and nurses, the expression on his face resembling medieval depictions of Saint Sebastian being pierced with arrows. Bellany and I became friends, and he gave me some lessons, especially in the use of color, of which he is a master. During one session, I had to paint Bellany himself, and I realized that my interpretation of a really sick man recovering from a major operation was very different from his.

Anatomical study has long been a joint focus for both artists and surgeons, but I am convinced that artists are unlikely to produce important works unless they are thoroughly trained in the basic tech-

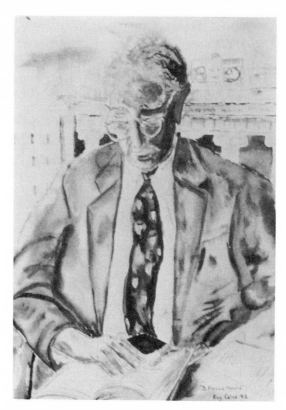

Sir Roy Calne, *A Patient Recovering from Operation*

niques of painting and unless they feel strongly about their subject matter. Emotions can be simulated, and in medical practice often are, but in art simulation is not enough, because the image must convey a message to the beholder without long explanatory notes or conversation.

In that regard, the American surgeon Rudolph Matas wrote: "In spite of the triple coat of mail with which the surgeon must often encase his heart, in order to accomplish his tasks successfully, he is, nevertheless, a man, a human, and as such he is unavoidably and most painfully affected by suffering and death when these overtake the young, the gentle and the beautiful."

That feeling of devastation comes to me almost inevitably, regardless of the age, disposition, or beauty of the patient who has sought my help. I am often haunted by the hopeful, trusting faces of relatives and patients for whom I have not done enough, no matter how desperate the situation before the operation. My former chief Lord Brock once remarked, "There is no question but that the sorrows and bitter moments in surgery can fade before the great and intense satisfaction that comes when a difficult problem has been brought safely to a happy conclusion." For me, painting distills the very essence of what Lord Brock was getting at, and I hope that in my work I testify to the witness of Rudolph Matas.

It also occurred to me that transplantation was a subject nobody had ever painted, because it did not exist apart from the legends of Saints Cosmos and Damian transplanting a leg in the Middle Ages. Moreover, I had models who were not only captive while patients in the hospital but often pleased at the chance of sitting, so that they could talk to the surgeon about little things he or she otherwise wouldn't have time for. In particular, I was able to become friends with children, who are usually terrified of doctors and nurses. But having the doctor sit down with a piece of paper and a pencil, and minus the white coat, immediately relaxes a child, who understands that this is going to be fun and won't hurt. I often give photocopies of the outline to the child so that both of us can paint it. This has enabled me to become friends with children and to understand some of their fears and their courage.

In past years I have painted many patients, adult and child; many colleagues—doctors, nurses, and scientists; the donors; and the operation itself (plate 1). Art has become a major activity. Some people ask me if I find it therapeutic; rather, I find it a challenge. As with the biology of transplantation, which we will never fully understand, one never paints as well as one would like. I have exhibited my works, especially at transplant meetings, to try to show the human side of transplantation, to encourage organ donation, and to increase public understanding of the process. Transplantation is not just a huge media event of an operation but a serious attempt to restore the life of a person doomed by ill health.

The coming together of surgery and art has for me been a satisfying, if sometimes frustrating and disappointing, experience. The challenge continues.

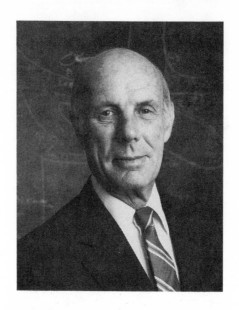

Our second painter, ERNEST CRAIGE, is a cardiologist with a gift for cartooning, a talent that proved invaluable to him first as a medical student and later as a teacher at the University of North Carolina at Chapel Hill. Humor is Craige's trademark; his first book of cartoons, an entertaining account of his World War II experiences in Europe, was widely acclaimed. Dr. Craige likes to use cartoons to warn the public about dangers to health, because "an ominous message is sometimes better received through humor than through fear." In retirement, he has found time to memorialize his travels in watercolors.

Making the Scene

Ernest Craige, M.D.

Webster's defines *afield* as "abroad" or "astray." To me, however, drawing and painting are intricately involved in the practice and teaching of medicine. I hope to illustrate that relationship here.

My decision to go into medicine was not difficult. My father was a pediatrician, much beloved by his patients and their families. I had to decide on a career in the depths of the Depression, and although I had been drawing since early childhood, I knew that earning a living with brush or pen would not be easy. On entering the University of North Carolina, I therefore chose the premedical curriculum.

In the mid-1930s, most institutions of higher learning encouraged, or at least tolerated, college humor magazines. These have almost all disappeared in today's more politically correct atmosphere. I soon became art editor of the *Carolina Buccaneer*, the school magazine, and found rich material for pen-and-ink cartoons in the hypocrisy of the fraternity system, the frenzied social weekends, and the eccentricities of the faculty. My editorship was unusually distinguished in that we were not banned from the mails for including lewd material.

My involvement in campus publications may have been a factor in receiving a Rhodes Scholarship in 1939. On the day I was scheduled to sail for England, however, Hitler launched his Polish campaign and the Oxford experience had to be scrapped. Instead, I went to Harvard Medical School (HMS), where my class participated in the abbreviated curriculum necessitated by the war. In medical school, drawing was a vital component of my note taking in anatomy, physiology, public health, and other courses. HMS published an annual volume that I illustrated using subject matter from our exciting clinical experiences, such as delivering babies in peoples' homes.

Harvard's senior play in 1943 was set on a remote South Pacific island, principally in a saloon called the Median Bar. This called for a barroom nude of large dimensions, an element of the scenery that I created and that was highly prized by the two classes that year. It was unfurled at every class reunion thereafter and finally this artistic work became part of the permanent collection at the Countway Library at Harvard, thus ensuring its availability to future generations!

Those who graduated from medical school in spring 1943 were inducted, after a brief internship, into the armed services. Some fifteen hundred other soldiers and I sailed for Glasgow on the *Queen Mary* in the summer of 1944. My group, an auxiliary surgical unit, worked in France, Belgium, Holland, and Germany. Fortunately, I had ample drawing supplies and so recorded many of the tragicomic events and people along our route. I soon became aware of the authorities' concern with venereal disease. (This, of course, was before penicillin, and the army camps were ringed by eager reservoirs of infection.) I responded to the challenge by producing a series of posters with such slogans as "Fools Rush in Where Angels Fear to Bed"; "Just 'Cause She's Demure, Don't Mean She's Pure"; and "Too Many Cooks Spoil the Brothel!"—though they were never used. Later, these drawings were privately published under the title *Our Hearts Were Young with Gay* (Gay was our commanding officer), copies of which were given to friends, classmates, and members of my outfit.

After the war, I completed house-staff training at Massachusetts General Hospital. It was my good fortune to fall under the direction of two outstanding clinicians and teachers, Paul D. White and Chester Jones. Dr. White had a profound knowledge of cardiology, as encapsulated in his classic textbook, *Heart Disease* (1931). He was remarkably thoughtful and appreciative of everyone from the cleaning person to the medical specialist. He could manage a consultation in a difficult case such that the referring physician was given credit for changes in treatment, to the satisfaction and relief of all concerned.

After a few years with Dr. White at Harvard, I was invited to join the faculty at the University of North Carolina at Chapel Hill, where the two-year school of medicine was being expanded to a full four years; in addition, a new hospital was under construction. The opportunity to build my own cardiology division in such ideal surroundings was irresistible.

Because the faculty in the early 1950s was minute (the Department of Medicine consisted of six people), each of us had an overwhelming array of duties. I soon found that in giving lectures and demonstrations, an easel and pastels were preferable to slides. A slide projector necessitates turning off the lights, a sure invitation to somnolence. Often the clutter of information on a slide is too formidable for an unprepared audience. It proved more effective to start with blank paper on an easel of the type used by traveling salesmen and explain a point through drawings. Pastels in brilliant colors and ample size (one-inch square in cross section) produce a mark easily visible in an amphitheater. By my starting with a blank sheet and building up an image, whether of an anatomical concept or of physiological events such as the cardiac cycle, the student could easily follow the progression of material and was often intrigued by the apparent spontaneity of the demonstration. In explaining the events of the cardiac cycle, for instance, I started with the electrocardiogram and added the pressure, volume, valvular, and auscultatory events in various pastel colors. These complex relationships could be sketched lightly in pencil over vertical time lines prior to the demonstration. This helped show the simultaneity of related events and avoided mistakes or omissions during a presentation.

The same technique lent itself to lectures for lay audiences. A cartoon created on the spot could demonstrate vividly how some individuals flirt with disaster through unhealthy diet, lack of exercise, smoking, and the like. An ominous message is sometimes better received through humor than through fear. Grand rounds, clinical pathological conferences, and other gatherings in medical school provided grist for cartoons and sketches that helped cement the point

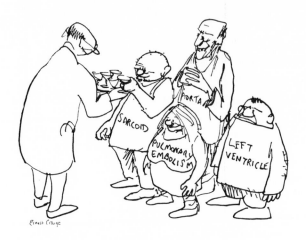

Ernest Craige, "Entertaining a Diagnosis"

under discussion—or perhaps provided diversion from a tedious presentation. Committee meetings, which could get out of hand timewise, furnished ample material for caricatures. The sketch pad, held at a discreet angle, can simulate note taking and thereby avoid giving offense. A cartoon entitled "Entertaining a Diagnosis" was inspired by one such meeting.

I have enjoyed providing illustrations for the *Harvard Medical Alumni Bulletin*, the *New England Journal of Medicine*, and the *Journal of the Swiss Medical Association*. I have also created Christmas and birthday cards and posters for community events such as Mardi Gras, which my daughters had a good time coloring.

My retirement in the mid-1980s brought free time and new opportunities. (I resisted the temptation of part-time teaching or patient care. A part-time cardiologist should be avoided, I think, for the same reasons one would want to avoid an occasional pilot of a 747!) My previous cartooning had principally been in black and white; the use of color had been postponed for lack of time. Success in realistic watercolors (as opposed to abstraction) calls for competence in drawing. In my case, some sixty years of drawing is probably more than should be recommended, but it preceded my plunge into color.

I found watercolor exhilarating. The equipment is simple, portable, and inexpensive, and the results are quickly obtained, to keep or discard. In the past ten years I have had four exhibitions and have sold scores of paintings (plates 2 and 3). Seeing my work in the homes of friends is extremely rewarding. I would happily distribute my paintings gratis, but I have learned that such gifts are not as well appreciated as paintings that one has personally selected and paid for. Like being in psychotherapy or playing poker, it doesn't do you any good until you put some of your own money into it!

I think of drawing and painting as a way of improving my powers of observation, of recording what I see, and of demonstrating and teaching. The process of distilling the essentials of a natural scene in nature or of the gesture of a dancer or laborer seems to me to bring the subject to life in the viewer's mind much more effectively than does a photographic essay. The hobby of art gives me a welcome respite from the stresses and cares of professional work. Attempting to create my own art greatly enhances my appreciation of the works of great masters as seen in museums. In the medical field, art can help not only in teaching but also in the therapeutic relief of stress and frustration (for patient and doctor alike).

Some people claim they can't draw a straight line. Fortunately, straight lines don't appear in nature, so I would advise carrying a sketchpad and pencil and trying your hand.

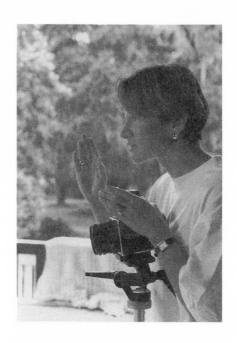

ANDREA BALDECK has led a remarkable life
because of her two afield activities: the French horn
and photography. Attracted by the practice of medicine in Third World countries such as Haiti and
Grenada, Baldeck left her job as an anesthesiologist in
the United States and went out into the world "to
capture and possibly make sense of it through the lens
of a camera." Her photographic interests are eclectic,
but her most recent collection has focused on the
Hôpital Albert Schweitzer in Haiti.

Life through the Lens

Andrea M. Baldeck, M.D.

A sense of adventure led me into the field of medicine, and beyond. Growing up in a farming village where the world was defined by silos and cornfields, I yearned for the faraway and the exotic, as seen in the local library's *National Geographic*s. Within these pages I found biographies written for children and became captivated by Albert Schweitzer. Here was someone with several careers, someone who had struck out for unknown Africa to deliver the most potent magic of all: medicine!

Those grainy black-and-white photographs stirred my imagination like nothing before. Here were lush Kipling-esque jungles and broad waterways where stately black men rowed dugout canoes to the landing below Schweitzer's hospital in Lambaréné, Gabon. Patients of all ages, with diseases I'd barely heard of, gathered at the clinic door. In the middle of all this was Schweitzer—tending to a gamut of ills all day, and by evening writing or sending the piano strains of Bach into the night. In the early 1950s *Life* produced a stunning photo essay on Dr. Schweitzer, a recent Nobel laureate, taken by the preeminent American photojournalist W. Eugene Smith. These images seized my imagination all those years ago—and continue to do so.

I was smitten! This was the career for me, combining travel to remote equatorial places and (to salve my Calvinistic conscience in the face of all this fun) the opportunity to do "good works" as a physician. The image of a local general practitioner diligently answering house calls with a Gladstone bag held no appeal; I felt sure that my life would be different. At age ten, one's notions of the future avoid the gravitational pull of reality.

I combed the library for more stories of adventurer-doctors and discovered Tom Dooley's medical exploits in Indochina and the signal accomplishments of Dr. Warren Seagraves, a surgeon in Burma. Poring over geographical atlases on wintry afternoons, I imagined myself in tropical settings far from my placid, ice-encrusted hometown.

Still, the lure of medicine competed with my interest in becoming a professional musician. Early piano lessons had yielded to eighteen years of studying the French horn. The joy of expression in sound, in both solo and ensemble playing, fired ambitions to play with a first-class orchestra. When this grandiose vision dimmed in early adulthood, my thoughts returned to the dream of medicine. I knew this field would be as demanding a taskmaster as music in its claims on time and energy, but it admitted diligent "section players" as well as virtuosi. Several years of work prepared me for my next "audition," and at age twenty-five I found myself in medical school. How exactly to reach the lands of my distant childhood imaginings presented more of a problem, as none of my peers or teachers seemed sympathetic to my vision. I placed my jungle doctor notions on the shelf, next to music, through the many years of schooling and apprenticeship that followed.

Well into a residency in internal medicine, I learned about the Hôpital Albert Schweitzer (HAS) in Haiti from someone who had been there years before. Haiti, though more accessible than Lambaréné, was just as mysterious to me, and I determined to spend some time at the hospital to test whether my childhood dreams could survive a firsthand experience. A year later, I found myself driving along the coast road north of Port-au-Prince in a jeep with a Haitian driver. To the left was the Caribbean; to the right, soaring, treeless mountains. Overhead, clouds threatened an afternoon storm so typical of the rainy season. Our route turned inland onto an unpaved road gouged with muddy potholes. Over the next two hours we bumped and splashed along, passing Haitians balancing large loads on their heads as they returned from fields and markets on foot or heavily laden donkeys; boisterous, barefoot children tagged alongside. By the time the jeep reached the hospital at the end of the road, I knew I was in for an adventure.

In the wards of the Hôpital Albert Schweitzer I encountered diseases I'd read about but had never treated. Many late nights were spent in the hospital library rereading texts that held new immediacy. (It's always humbling when your secretary recognizes diseases more quickly than you do.) I came away from that trip to Haiti with photographically sharp mental images that are still powerful in my memory: a gaunt young man, short of breath, eyes feverish with advanced tuberculosis, was a living picture of the "galloping consumption" of nineteenth-century novels. One afternoon a distraught father brought in his child, rigid as a board with tetanus. A spectral twenty-five-year-old arrived when the voodoo cure had failed: a bewildering series of infections, followed by lymphoma, rapidly brought on his death and gave a face to AIDS before it had a name. One stifling day during the rainy season a young woman with malaria, awaiting her turn to be seen, lay on the cold concrete floor to relieve her fever.

Haiti affected me profoundly. I returned home feeling that I'd gained more than I'd given and that my youthful notion of practicing medicine afield was truly possible. I traveled twice more to Haiti and once to Grenada with Project Hope. Each venture brought its challenges and dilemmas, but each return to the United States was increasingly difficult. Reentering a medical setting rife with waste, costly heroics, and defensive medical practice became harder and harder.

Vacations provided a chance to venture farther abroad—to Kilimanjaro, the Himalayas, the Atlas Mountains of Morocco—and to cast off for little-known islands. The camera was my constant companion, a means of capturing the faces and places that defined these disparate experiences. What I chose to photograph gradually revealed to me what I had not yet admitted to myself. While practicing medicine in the Western world, I longed for an assignment in the Third World; yet, even in the overflowing clinics of that world, I longed for yet more distant locales. There was no lack of satisfaction in delivering health care where it was so acutely needed, but working within the confines of a hospital one can receive the skewed impression that everyone in the society is ill. I wanted to go beyond those walls, to move about in a culture not my own, to interact with people outside the doctor-patient relationship and visually record their lives.

With each return from medical work or holiday in some far-flung locale, I found the operating suite of an urban medical center increasingly suffocating. The fluorescent-lit, windowless rooms were effectively a sterile microcosm within the hospital. Despite the intense and rewarding work, I felt a growing sense of visual deprivation and a longing to experience a larger world. My appetite for adventure fired a desire to catch the magic of the instant in photographs, like insects in amber.

When the opportunity arose, I left anesthesiology to pursue the medium of black-and-white photography, apprenticing myself to a friend and professional in the field. With the acquisition of suitable cameras and the construction of a darkroom, my long residency in photography began. One of my first humbling lessons was learning just how much time and film are needed to arrive at worthwhile images. As in medicine and music, the art and science of the discipline demand attention and diligent practice. My respect for the human retina and occipital cortex grew when I perceived how much more limited was the recording medium of photographic emulsion. Whereas the brain takes a high-resolution image and edits it with lightning speed to make the best sense of it for the conscious mind, the camera is, for all its refinements, a light-gathering box that simply records the rays that fall through the lens onto the film. Frequently the results reflect the lack of thought on the part of the operator.

To photograph is to manipulate light over finite time, using the physics of optics. This is not some mantra that the beginning photographer recites to achieve a higher awareness; nonetheless, to work with a camera is to become acutely aware of light in all its nuances. In black-and-white photography, the spectrum is translated into a scale of grays bounded by white and black. In the absence of color, the play of light and shadow remains; these forces have been integral to the art and belief systems of humankind for millennia. The relationships and structures of the picture—its anatomy—stand out in relief. The image is abstracted from our multihued reality, yet at the same time a moment, an emotion, or a message can powerfully assert itself in the absence of color's distraction.

Here the sensibility of the photographer comes into play, in a hunt for subject matter best suited to the medium. This search becomes continuous and unconscious, whether or not a camera is in hand, because it becomes a way of seeing, a highly attuned visual awareness. The challenge is to transfer what the mind's eye sees to the two-dimensional sheet of photographic paper.

Merely bringing that image into being engaged much of my attention as a beginning photographer. Wielding a camera is much like playing a musical instrument: both are tools for expression. To successfully execute a composition requires technical proficiency, the ability to recognize and articulate interrelationships within it, and sensitivity to timing and tonality. Steady practice—engaging eyes, ears, and hands—hones the senses and develops the muscle memory needed to express an idea *through* the instrument rather than in spite of it. Early on, before my responses with the camera became internalized and reflexive, many wrong notes and visual dissonances rang out from practice rolls. Occasionally, ensnared by a technical question, I would find that my subject had run off or that daylight had faded while I pondered my choices.

Was all this studious self-application necessary? I wondered. Most of the world seemed satisfied with the point-and-shoot approach. Yet the more I studied the work of notable photographers, the more I came to appreciate that most great photographs are made with vision and a large share of hard-earned skill, occasionally enhanced with a touch of luck. Every frame represents an opportunity to record a meaningful subject in what Ansel Adams calls the "perfect negative," a way of translating the evanescence of time and light into the permanence of silver salts suspended in emulsion.

Of course, darkroom chemistry must fix these grains of silver permanently before one can hold the negative up to the light with an appraising squint. Any resemblance to rapid photo processing vanishes during the task of turning a carefully selected negative into an enlarged print. Hours can elapse while exposure time, contrast control, and development are fine-tuned to produce a print that re-creates what the eye saw when the shutter clicked. If after five hours three prints emerge from the darkroom to face the light of day and the scrutiny of others, the time has been well spent. When I leave the darkroom after hours in the twilight glow of a safelight, it seems ironic that, to produce a record of what was seen in the light, I must work in the dark. Having left the windowless operating room, I now work in a windowless darkroom but find that the creative tensions in the latter are far preferable to the white-knuckle scenes in the former; in the darkroom, if you make a mistake, no one dies.

When a physician is introduced to a new acquaintance, the inevitable question seems to be, "And what is your specialty?" This question is also asked of photographers: Is it landscape, portraiture, architectural subjects? Are the results destined for commercial or fine-art markets? At first, any subject is fair game; quantities of film are consumed in just getting it right. As time goes on, one gravitates to particular interests or challenges.

I take pictures of people: not the stolen or grab shots of the photojournalist or the furtive tourist, or the portraits of the mall studio, but those requiring direct engagement with the subject in situ—situational portraits where the setting adds depth to the subject. Summoning up the courage to approach a stranger and asking that person to be a subject is one of those risky ventures whose outcome is rarely predictable: the occasional surprises reveal as much about the photographer as about the subject. I still steel myself during these encounters, though I no longer feel like a novice. An invitation by the gallery owner Helen Drutt to photograph several world-renowned craft artists provided an opportunity to polish my portrait technique. She had a limited budget and expansive ideas, but I was happy to work for the experience alone. We wanted to show the artists in their studios and to reveal how the work that emerged was inextricably linked to the personality of the maker and the space where it was made.

Most memorable was our encounter with an octogenarian ceramist with an international reputation for crafting translucent vessels from his secret formula for porcelain. With snowy hair and beard, lively blue eyes, a gently taciturn manner, and a spartan lifestyle, Rudi Staffel on first meeting resembled an Amish farmer more than a revered artist. His rowhouse studio in a nineteenth-century industrial neighborhood was a still life of dusty disarray. Bags of wet and dry ingredients, mixing tools, and notebooks splattered with dried globs of porcelain lay in one corner. Potential subject matter—dead flowers in dusty vases, an odd jar, an old photograph—sat in the gloomy light that straggled in through streaked windowpanes.

Amid it all Rudi was putting the finishing touches on a bowl, and a unique object of beauty emerged from its inchoate surroundings. I realized that he was, with remarkably successful results, husbanding his energies for the creative act rather than the cleanup. Other finished pieces, occupying a display shelf draped in black felt, looked chalky and opaque until Rudi switched on the bulb above them, bringing them to life in their otherworldly translucence. Somehow, not only order but elegance had been distilled out of chaos.

A visual equivalent of this paradigm came together in a series of photographs. With Rudi's approval and Helen's efforts, they appeared in the museum catalogue for his fifty-year retrospective in Helsinki. Greatly enlarged, they became part of the installation itself. As the show and its catalogue travel to other museums, they provide a validation of my work, of the direction I have taken since leaving medicine. My recurrent misgivings since that departure have been quieted, letting me move forward more confidently in my new field.

Five years after changing careers, an invitation to photograph at the Hôpital Albert Schweitzer provided an opportunity to integrate several strands of my experience. It had been eleven years since my last tour of duty there, and much had happened in Haiti: the flight of "Baby Doc" Duvalier; the election, overthrow, and exile of Father Aristide; the economic embargo by the Organization of American States; refugee flotillas of desperate boat people; bloody civil unrest; the brokered departure of the oppressive General Raoul Cedras; peaceful occupation by the U.S. Marines, and the joyous return of President Aristide. My anticipation grew as travel plans were finalized; on the day of my departure, I boarded a flight to Port-au-Prince in Miami, shouldering my camera equipment and one hundred rolls of film. All around me were the Creole conversations of homeward-bound Haitians, some visiting from their expatriate enclaves in Montreal and New York, others hoping to start a new life in the more hopeful political and economic climate.

Stepping off the plane in the torrid Haitian afternoon, I felt as if I had never been away. In the arrivals terminal was the familiar maelstrom of distracted travelers, porters muscling bulging suitcases and duct-taped cardboard cartons, hyperkinetic taxi drivers competing for fares, and gesticulating friends and families straining at the barriers for a glimpse of those long awaited. Amid this chaos I located the driver sent for me by the hospital, and we threaded our way to the HAS jeep.

Our route out of the capital skirted one of its fetid slums, grown larger and grimmer in the embargo years, and then plunged us into the cacophonous traffic of a Friday afternoon. It was Good Friday, and traffic was repeatedly halted by the celebrants of RaRa, a Lenten spectacle begun in colonial times when plantation owners granted their slaves brief leave to visit those on other plantations. This revelry, once the clever pretext for keeping genetic diversity in the workforce, remains alive in boisterous parades that guarantee impromptu costumes, percussion and horns, and liberal measures of rum. A normally long trip out to the bush grew longer and longer. Sunset was approaching as we entered the relative calm of the hospital compound, and I felt as if I had come home. I was welcomed by Mrs. Gwen Mellon, the indomitable eighty-five-year-old director of the hospital, which she had founded with her late husband, Dr. Larry Mellon, in 1956.

Over the next ten days I came to know the hospital far better than during my longer previous stays, when work confined me to clinic, wards, and operating room. Now I ventured far beyond the compound to document the hospital's outreach to the two hundred thousand inhabitants of the Artibonite River Valley. Daily forays on rutted roads with an intrepid driver and various hospital staff—a Haitian physician, health aides, a veterinarian, a Mennonite teacher-trainer—provided a wide-angle view of Haitian life on rural farms and in market villages. At a hospital-supported dispensary, a straw-hatted mother stood under the trees and hugged her infant, who was there to be immunized against tetanus, long a scourge here. Among mud-and-wattle huts with roofs of thatched cornhusks, a health worker visited a patient with advanced AIDS and conferred with the extended family about terminal care. Small children mugged for the camera and one, diving into a hut, reappeared with a prized possession —a much worn magazine photo of Titid, President Aristide. Flood and drought exact their price in the valley, and the lack of potable water promotes typhoid and other enteric infections, which claim the youngest and oldest. We left our truck on the riverbank to speak with a work team repairing a vital irrigation dam for control of flow to surrounding rice paddies. Miles down another dirt road, women gathered in a church with a simple earthen floor. After a day spent selling in the market and caring for their families, they sat expectantly, workbooks in hand, before their teacher in literacy class. They would work until dusk and dinner called them home.

With my battered porkpie hat and two cameras, I moved among the people, trying to portray their spirit, their dignity, their hard work, and the inevitability of their death. I could not be unobtrusive: blending into the background and catching my subjects unawares was not an option. I had to explain myself constantly—sometimes through an interpreter, often in my limited Creole—and to ask permission to photograph my subjects. Many agreed to participate when told that the project was to benefit their hospital, not to generate profits for myself in a distant commercial market. From them I learned that when you feel that all you possess is your own image, it is given sparingly and with gravity, as the most personal of gifts.

After days in the countryside, dreams of scenes and faces crowded my sleep. I awoke hoping that these images were not mere wraiths of memory but also truths awaiting me in photographic emulsion. Not until weeks later (a month of which I spent in the clutches of *Giardia*) would two thousand negatives emerge from the darkroom into daylight. These, transferred onto stacks of contact sheets, demanded careful editing to the point of nystagmus. With grease pencil posed above the thumb-sized images, I outlined frames for future scrutiny, only a fraction of which would merit enlargement. The first month yielded photographs needed for immediate use by the hospital— personnel, places, projects—for newsletters, brochures, and archives. Then I began to print the faces that most vividly colored my memories of Haiti. They represented for me all those who make the Artibonite Valley their home and call the Hôpital Albert Schweitzer their hospital. In their expressions appeared the strength, resilience, and spirit of the Haitian people, who conduct their lives with dignity and season their talk with proverbs such as "Si ou pa lion, fe ou réna" (If you're not a lion, be a fox); "Fanm sé kajou: plus li vié, plus li bon"

(Woman is mahogany tree: more she's old, more she's good); and "Kréyon Bon Dié pa gin gonm" (God's pencil has no eraser).

When spread out on a long wooden table (made of Antillean oak in Haiti), the forty strongest photographs began to suggest a book, primarily of images rather than of text, that would reveal a Haiti not seen in newspapers or on television screens. The directness of the subjects' gazes demanded equally powerful captions. Haitian proverbs in Creole and English were matched with the photographs. A simple title fit the contents: *The Heart of Haiti*.

No sooner was the darkroom work complete than months of work with the book designer and printer began; I learned the logistics behind a volume of fine-art photography. The original prints were rephotographed in separate negatives to make the lithographic plates for the press. Critical choices of layout, typeface, paper, and ink contributed to the desired effect. Each proof was checked for problems as it came off the drum of the press—a process that can take weeks. Even at this stage, the finished book seemed far removed from the stacks of uncut sheets at the press. Only when the mockup from the bindery arrived did the book feel fully real. More time elapsed before a delivery truck unloaded box after box of shrink-wrapped bound volumes.

As my gift to HAS in its fortieth year, most of this press run went directly to the stateside foundation that supports the hospital. By now the book has reached friends of the hospital in North America, Europe, and Haiti and has accompanied an exhibit of the original prints in Philadelphia. Mrs. Mellon has given copies to the heads of Haitian government, and a New York publisher has voiced interest in a trade edition. As the prints travel to regional museums and galleries, it is my hope that the work will speak to a wide audience and will add to the photographic legacy of rural Haiti produced by the likes of Eugene Smith and Walter Rosenblum.

My involvement with Haiti continues, but I have also pursued other photographic avenues, involving new techniques and ways of seeing. As with medicine, photography provides multiple possibilities: for specialization, for ongoing learning, and for exploring the instruments available to the eye and hand.

One such instrument is the large-format camera, which has

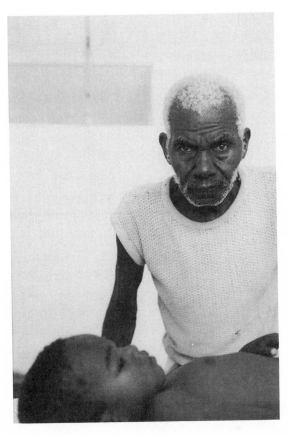

Andrea Baldeck, *Tiger Old but Claws Never Old*
(Creole proverb)

changed little over the last century. Many of our forebears posed before this machine; its bellows and lens transmit an inverted image onto a ground-glass screen. Under a black cloth, the photographer crouches to compose the frame and adjust the focus. The postures and solemn expressions assumed by the subjects were a result of the slow film and shutter speeds. Although faster film has reduced some of these constraints, the subject matter must still be tailored to the instrument. With the large-format camera, one forgoes the quick, candid frame for the deliberate, disciplined shot. What limits the versatility of this camera—its size—is also its strength, for it can produce a page-sized negative of exquisite detail. Thus equipped, Ansel Adams documented Yosemite to stunning effect, while Edward Weston transformed two peppers into a sensuous abstract study. In hopes of creating still lifes worthy of this camera, I build small altars draped in black to hold talismanic subject matter gathered from the natural world.

The large-format camera also shares characteristics of the French horn I played for so many years: its bulk, its commanding presence, and the physical demands it makes of its operator. For subtlety, lightness, and ease of transport, I choose the flute and the 35-mm camera, the two of which slip easily into a camera bag.

At the cost of producing a smaller negative, the 35-mm photographer gains mobility, speed, and unlimited shooting locations. The secret scenes of Henri Cartier-Bresson, the portraits of Sebastião Salgado, and the humor of Elliot Erwitt come to mind as I venture into the avenues of Paris, the winding waterways of Venice, the dusty lanes of a remote island village, or my own backyard. Anything within reach of the camera becomes fair game: this is what continues to lure photographers out of the studio and into the world. Does such activity generate a greater understanding for the world? Not necessarily. But the failure to venture out and engage the mind and senses inevitably teaches nothing.

The prospect of adventure, and of acquiring skills, has drawn me to medicine, music, and photography. Medicine probes the internal complexities of the organism, using compassionate science to restore and regenerate the human mind and corpus. Music speaks convincingly in a language that transcends words. Photography molds the qualities of light to illuminate the visual complexity of life. Each métier provides a way of ordering perceptions, suggests interrelationships of the parts to form a whole, and tantalizes with the promise of discovery and understanding. At the center of all three is the search, with mind and senses in pursuit of a satisfying resolution—a diagnosis, a closing cadence, or a perfect print. Both art and medicine demand of their practitioners sensitivity and long-term commitment; both have restorative, healing effects. Their striking similarities aside, however, the powers vested in each differ: for while medicine can cure the body, art can cure the soul.

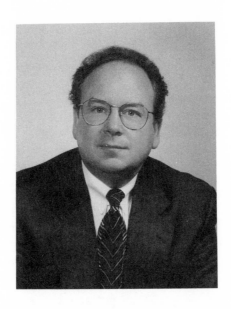

MARK H. SWARTZ tells us of his rigorous teaching program at Mount Sinai School of Medicine and of a daily schedule so demanding that involvement in an activity outside medicine seems an impossibility. Dr. Swartz has originated a new form of photography—known as Photodigitography—by manipulating photographs through digital imaging. These entrancing new visual experiences have been widely exhibited and acclaimed; one of his pictures hangs in the White House. An innovative teacher as well, he trains students at Mount Sinai to become better doctors by simulating doctor-patient interactions using professional actors. It is no surprise that Dr. Swartz's bedtime is 2:45 A.M. and that he rises only a few hours later to be at the hospital by 7:30.

Letting Colors Dance

Mark H. Swartz, M.D.

Teaching physical diagnosis for the past twenty years has taught me the principle of inspection — the ability to use my vision to understand the world better. My eye has been trained to look closely at a subject and to see beyond the superficial characteristics. This clinical skill has allowed me to see the world more clearly and to frame my images through the camera with that same critical vision. There is so much a clinician and photographer have in common—the ability, as Sir William Osler said, "to teach the eye to see."

One of my typical days at the hospital includes conferring with colleagues, lecturing to students, and seeing patients. Finally, at around 10 P.M., I can relax, sit down at my computer, and begin to transform photographs. Using a high-tech computer-graphics system, I am able to take a portion of a prosaic scene and make it colorful, complex, and sometimes surreal. Blue dances with orange and fades into shades of purple. A simple white calla lily becomes a pale lavender pastel study with yellow and green highlights; a pure white Easter lily becomes a dazzling burst of iridescent hues resembling stained glass; a saxophonist in a Stockholm marching band is reconstituted into colored specks resembling pointillistic brush strokes.

From the beginning, my career in medicine left little time for my other passion: photography. In 1969, after graduating from college, I was among the first students at the new Mount Sinai School of Medicine. Photography had to wait on the sidelines. While in medical school, I married Vivian Hirshaut, my college sweetheart, who was attending the Albert Einstein College of Medicine. The small apartment we rented near Mount Sinai had no space for a darkroom. In 1973, Vivian began postgraduate training in ophthalmology, and I in internal medicine and cardiology. In 1977, we moved into a house in Westchester County, which allowed me to set up a darkroom and experiment with color and image.

After becoming an academic cardiologist, I had opportunities to travel and teach in many countries. My camera was always ready—I might take as many as fifteen hundred shots in two weeks. I focused on simple things, not necessarily "picture postcards" of the scenery. A blade of grass breaking through an old Roman amphitheater in Israel or a dew drop on a flower in Thailand might attract my attention. On returning, I processed all the film myself, and some of my better shots won national and international awards. One image, of two men praying at the Western wall in Jerusalem, appeared on the cover of *Life* magazine in the early 1980s. Despite an exhausting day at Mount Sinai, most evenings find me in the darkroom experimenting with photographic techniques.

In 1989, I published the *Textbook of Physical Diagnosis: History and Examination,* with an emphasis on humanistic medicine. That volume became a turning point in both my academic and photographic careers, for it led me to head a medical teaching program at Mount Sinai Medical Center—the Morchand Center for Clinical Competence. Dedicated to training today's medical students to become tomorrow's compassionate physicians, the center's motto is a quotation from Hippocrates: "Where there is love for mankind, there is love for the art of healing." More than one hundred of my photos were chosen to hang on the walls of the reception area and examination rooms. The Morchand Center attracted visitors from around the country, many of whom wanted to buy my photographs. Buy *my* photographs? I had never publicly shown or sold any of them. I began to inquire about galleries, and thus my career as an artist was launched.

That same year, I was accepted for membership in an art gallery in Westchester, New York. After several group shows, the gallery director called to say that the CEO of a large company in Beverly Hills had purchased my "Speckled Lily" for his office. I was amazed and overjoyed that someone wanted to own my work.

But I wanted to do something different. My love for photography and my interest in computers were now coming together. At first, I used a store-bought photo-editing program to scan images into the computer, but then I began to write my own programs. With these programs, I would like to think that I have achieved unique enhancements of photographs, which differ from other computer-manipulated works. Although I check off "Photography," "Graphic Arts," or "Fine Art" on entry forms for art shows, my style of work fits none of these categories.

I call this art form Photodigitography. Through digital imaging and photography, the most ordinary subject matter can become something entirely new. I select a 35-mm color slide, scan it into the computer, alter the image using my programs, create a new film original, and finally produce a Cibachrome print, a positive-to-positive process for producing archival-quality prints in the conventional darkroom. In my darkroom, I can make Cibachrome prints up to sixteen by twenty inches.

In the past I had to travel around the globe for subjects, but now they are right at hand, within one hundred feet of my darkroom: for example, lilies, azaleas, cosmos, and roses from our garden, even our pet parakeet and cat. Single flowers, parts of animal faces, became abstract and unrecognizable. Over the years, I have accumulated over eighty-five thousand images of people, scenes, still lifes, carnivals, fireworks, nudes, flowers, and hot-air balloons, all subjects that can be used to create new images. In 1993, "Inside Ballooning" won first prize from among more than six thousand entries in the 1993 Artfolio International Art Competition.

On May 15, 1994, my first one-man show opened, with a preview that day in the *New York Times*. More than seven hundred people attended. Nearly all fifty-four pieces in the show sold, many several times over. I received orders for pieces to be enlarged, some up to four by six feet! I was now getting commissions. My fondest memory of that show occurred one evening at the gallery. A sick-looking man about thirty-five years old wandered in, looked around, and approached me to purchase two of the works. He had been feeling par-

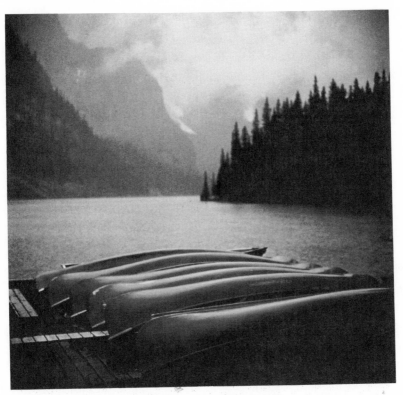

Mark Swartz, *Moraine Lake*

ticularly low-spirited, he told me, as the result of a three-week hospitalization. He was driving home when he saw the brilliant colors in the gallery window. He said my art had cheered him so much that he had to buy some for his home. My art had become a form of therapy!

Since then, I have had many shows, and my work is now in many private and corporate collections. "The Saxophonist" is part of President and Mrs. Clinton's private collection at the White House. In 1994, one of my nonmanipulated images, "Moraine Lake," was chosen out of thirty-three thousand entries as a winner in *American Photo*'s annual photographic contest. Shot on a rainy day near Lake Louise in the Canadian Rockies, the icy-green water and the red canoes in the foreground are visually exciting, but at the same time they have a strongly calming effect. As a four-by-four-foot enlargement, this image hangs in the waiting rooms of several psychiatrists.

Their patients have mentioned coming in early for appointments just to look at the vista and relax.

One of my favorite images is entitled "Siri." This was originally an image of an iris, significantly enlarged and turned upside down. A reviewer in *Manhattan Arts International* wrote of "Siri" (iris spelled backward), "The abstracted forms, fragmented colors and sharply demarcated delineations throughout the picture exude a robust symphony of textures and tones in perpetual motion."

My passion for hot-air ballooning has often brought me to the Albuquerque International Balloon Fiesta, where I have sometimes served as an official photographer. Some of my favorite shots have been taken while floating through the air. The cover story of *Silver Kris,* the in-flight magazine of Singapore Airlines, described the transformation of one of these images, an example of which is "To Fly" (plate 4). Over the years, reviewers in the *New York Times, Artsnews,* and *Diversion* have generously termed my work "other-worldly," "a pure celebration of nature, color and technology," "expressionistic," and "stunning, displaying a sophisticated grasp of composition and form."

After focusing for so long on children, animals, and flowers, I changed venues a bit by developing an educational exhibit that centered on images of hatred, pain, and loss. "Faces of the Holocaust" debuted in Manhattan in March 1996. The exhibit consisted of twenty-five montages produced by photodigitography, based on photographs acquired by my father-in-law after his imprisonment during the Holocaust. One reviewer stated, "The product defies description. Filtering photography's hard evidence through the computer's unemotional overlay, the results jar like clashing notes sustained in unison." This exhibit has toured museums around the country.

I am often asked if I plan to give up medicine and devote all my time to photography. The answer is no. I need both to maintain my balance. Perhaps my love for photography has allowed me to see things more clearly or, as Osler observed, has taught my eye to see. It has certainly given me an escape from the daily anxieties of being a cardiologist and teacher. I'm glad to have both careers.

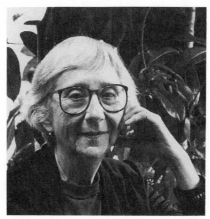

Penny Harris

BARBARA YOUNG, a psychiatrist, provides us
with insight into how her afield work has influenced
her medical career and how photography has
complemented her life as a psychiatrist. Creativity is
the link: photography can penetrate the mystery of
human beings and the process of becoming. Her
thoughtful essay emphasizes how the creative eye
opens new vistas into the heart—both hers and those
of the people she encounters each day.

In the Mind's Eye

MERGING VISIONS

Barbara Young, M.D.

My house on Herring Run in Baltimore is a working home. Patients wait in a living room; I have an office on the second floor; and my computer, the heart of my business activities, is next to my bed. But my home is also a showcase for my photographs: the walls are covered with pictures I have taken, and every nook and cranny is filled with negatives, slides, and enlargements.

"Painting with a camera" has been an ideal complement to my sedentary life as a psychiatrist. Not only does the camera get me outdoors, but it directs my energies away from the mental demands of listening to patients and helping them make sense of their lives.

When I told a doctor friend that I had combined the experiences of my two professions into a talk entitled "The Creative Way of Life," he asked, "Are you ambidextrous?" (I am.) He had come to the conclusion that those who are ambidextrous have more connections than other people between the right and left frontal cortex. Into my mind suddenly flashed an image of multicolored braids of yarn arching from one convoluted landscape to another. Here, perhaps, was an explanation for why I have become who I am. The tangling of those overabundant cables has been vexing at times, but they may have made it possible for me to work as both a doctor and an artist.

My parents were the first to direct me toward becoming a doctor. I was born in 1920, into a poor minister's family in rural Illinois. I believe my father must have wanted a doctor in our family. His brother Myron had practiced as a country doctor in Center Junction, Iowa. On occasional trips to his farm we enjoyed visiting his office, filled with bottles of colored pills that looked like candy; we licked our lips at the "tonic" he prescribed for us. (Did my father know it contained wine?)

My path toward medicine proceeded in barely perceptible steps. When I was only four or five, my family was standing on the porch of the parsonage in Brimfield, saying good-bye to relatives. Someone asked my brother Arthur what he wanted to be when he grew up. He emphatically declared, "I'm going to be a butcher!" I cried out, "I'm going to be a nurse!" To which grandmother replied, "But why don't you be a doctor?" Dear Mutty, my mother's mother—always to the rescue. Her input was unusual for 1925, but she and my grandfather were well acquainted with missionary doctors, both male and female. By the time I was an adolescent I also knew I did *not* want to be a teacher or a household drudge, for I sensed my intelligent, artistic mother's resentment of a life of service to her family.

When I was seventeen, my brother Harvey brought home *The Dissociation of a Personality,* by the psychologist Morton Prince. Up until that time, our early bedtime stories had been Sherlock Holmes; we reveled in the macabre adventures of Miss Beauchamp and her alter ego, Sally. That New Year's Eve I was reading alone, and terror seized me when I realized that a mind could split and war with itself. Dr. Prince had decreed that Sally must disappear. In furious rebellion, she forced Miss Beauchamp to stand in front of a mirror and "see" that her feet had been cut off, that all that remained were bloody stumps. This image was especially traumatic for me.

My adolescent years were painful; I was different from my classmates and friends. Fortunately, beginning in junior high, there was always at least one teacher who bolstered my self-confidence and flagging self-worth. I eventually discovered music, which sustained me and made life worthwhile; in junior high, I was the only cellist at the Knox College Conservatory. Sometime before high school graduation, I approached my physics teacher, Mr. Aitchison, and asked if he believed I could really become a doctor. My heart seemed to stop as he hesitated. No doubt he was taking into account my family's financial situation as well as my being a girl. Wise as he was, he knew how profoundly discouragement would have affected me. Kindly, he responded, "Yes, Barbara, I *think* you could be a doctor."

I entered Knox College in Galesburg, Illinois, as a premed major. In high school, I had found studying onerous and felt most at home in English classes, preferring *David Copperfield* to my geography textbook. *The Ambassadors,* by Henry James, proved especially meaningful to me: the protagonist, Strether, arrives in Paris to rescue his employer's son from a life of "indolence" but begins to question the value of his own life of toil and obedience and comes to believe in self-fulfillment as a worthy goal.

In my junior year of college Dr. Clarence Furrow encouraged me to visit medical schools. On these trips my evaluations were primarily intuitive: the sky over Northwestern University seemed heavy, for instance, and I sensed rigidity, authoritarianism. Weekly exams tested the students on each and every detail of their course work. Female students, observed a visiting physician, were expected to work all night long and be in the operating room early the next morning —with the seams of their stockings straight.

The atmosphere at the University of Chicago was the most congenial, and concepts were more important than details. My uncle, Arthur DeBra, visiting from New York, urged me to try Johns Hopkins as well; at the time I was not even aware that the university *had* a medical school. When a letter arrived from Hopkins offering me a half-tuition scholarship, I went to Baltimore with alacrity, even though the idea of becoming a doctor felt totally unreal. I was sure I had put one over on everyone—I could not possibly do the work required, nor did I have any driving desire to do so. I primarily wanted to escape from Galesburg and my fundamental unhappiness. Perhaps back East I would find a world where I belonged.

Baltimore was an oven when I arrived in June 1942, but I was so excited to be entering my "Paris" that I hardly noticed. I was welcomed with open arms at 800 North Broadway, familiarly known as the "Hen House." There, at long last, I discovered a group of young women just like me.

How to condense three of my happiest years into a few words? Because of the war, we covered four academic years in three by shortening the summer break. But time remained for walks in the park and weekend hikes to the quarries, where we swam in the cold water and sunned on the rocks. Our class came to feel like an extended family: we lived in small groups rather than large dormitories, and we were not informed of our course grades, reducing the sense of direct competition. The fellows at the anatomy table became our brothers.

Hopkins, like the University of Chicago, believed in the importance of understanding concepts rather than in the memorization of details. Tests were rare, and in this looser environment intimate conversation in the evening sometimes took precedence over books—we could study later. Anatomy, neuroanatomy, and physiology were easy to understand. The highest hurdle was chemistry, which two of the eight young women students were unable to surmount.

At Hopkins I did enjoy one brief moment of glory. A professor took several students to the bed of a patient and asked us to examine the man's heart. Each of the men percussed carefully. Concluding that the heart was enlarged, they drew lines at essentially the same place on the man's chest. When my turn came, I noticed a faint blue smudge in the axilla, the slightest dullness extending to that mark. Nervously I presented my findings to the professor, and it turned out that I was on the right track, for the patient had a huge pericardial effusion. That coup won me considerable esteem. This triumph has amused me ever since, for it had nothing to do with being a "good" doctor. My sensitive eye had come to my rescue. Someone once said of my photographs, "Barbara sees things we don't see." I can imagine no higher praise.

I had my first real experience as a doctor during my senior year, when I substituted for several weeks as a medical and surgical intern. The responsibilities, the gratification, the occasional disappointment, even the guilt that comes with the profession, all became real. I enjoyed working with patients but wished I could talk with them more. It was a heady experience, with no time to relax. Being on call day and night was deadly. I began to wonder if practicing medicine was how I wanted to spend the rest of my life. I envisioned years of great reward but constant exhaustion. I wanted to marry and have a family. Perhaps in psychiatry I would have more control of my time. On the fringe of my consciousness was an awareness that I needed time to discover and explore my own creative impulses if I was ever to be happy.

My love for psychiatry grew slowly. Our first exposure to the subject in medical school involved a handout, giving sketches of patients with their presenting symptoms and vignettes of their childhood experiences. The task of figuring out a diagnosis baffled many but seemed simple to me. In my fourth year I tried my hand at psychotherapy.

During my internship with a number of psychiatric patients, I attempted to understand what lay beneath their symptoms and how to further their personal growth.

In 1951 I started a private practice in Baltimore and continued my training in psychoanalysis at the Baltimore Psychoanalytic Institute. Today, after having worked as a psychiatrist for fifty years, I can honestly say that I have ended up exactly where I belong. I have thoroughly enjoyed my professional life and continue to do so.

At age thirty-six, in 1956, the sky went gray again. I was felled with repeated infections and forced to face the fact that something in my life was seriously out of balance. I followed Henry James's advice: "The tenement's haunted. Go abroad." Taking twelve weeks off, I sailed for Europe. While swimming in the Mediterranean, I was thrown against the rocks. Words sprang to mind—I had begun to write my first visual psychological sketch, "How Much Battering Can a Body Stand?" With this emergence of my artistic energies, the sky cleared for me and the world was joyful for the first time since my childhood.

Later I went to the Bahamas to write. My photographer brother, Arthur, had given me a Brownie camera. When he saw my first snapshots, he declared, "Barbara, you've got the eye! But you need a better camera." I had had no idea of my artistic ability. Soon I was "painting" seriously with the camera, working mostly in color; nature scenes gave way to architectural details. In the Bahamas I photographed people as a public service, since mine was the only camera in the village. Later *The Plop-a-Lop Tree,* my documentation of that Harbour Island community, was published.

Early on, my work met with good fortune. In 1961 Edward Steichen selected my *Golden Leaves* for the permanent collection of the

Museum of Modern Art in New York. In 1994 Richard Field, curator of the Yale University Art Gallery, accepted a series of images. Of numerous exhibitions over thirty-five years, the dearest to me have been in my current hometown. The Walters Art Gallery in Baltimore chose my photographs of Greece to accompany sculptures from their collection for a show entitled "The Ancient Greek World" in 1970. And in 1996 the Baltimore Museum of Art displayed some of my images among the work of others from my private collection in "A Photographer's Vision: Gifts to the Collection from Barbara Young."

For years I pursued photography at night, on weekends, and twice a year on vacations. As I grew older and wanted more time for photography and writing, I reduced my office hours. My life had largely involved "doing unto others," yet I began to feel more of a need to "do unto myself."

At times of crisis, taking pictures has been healing. When I was forty-five, I read my gynecologist's alarmed face during my annual pelvic exam. He had found a huge cyst that appeared to be malignant. With two weeks to get my house in order, to prepare patients for the possibility of going on without me, and to hang two photography shows, I had little time to be afraid. Postoperatively I awoke to the news that the cyst was endometrial but that a hysterectomy had been necessary. Six months later, in the Bahamas, I became engrossed in photographing two trees—one evergreen, one deciduous—whose outermost twigs interlaced above me. As I crawled on hands and knees trying to capture this "kiss," I began to shake. I realized that, for me, these trees symbolized a kiss of death. Not until then had I faced the close call I had had. The camera helped me with a necessary step in my full appreciation of life.

Pain itself cannot make an artist great. The gift of creativity must be inborn. I believe that all children are creative as long as their interests and skills are nourished. And childhood pain, if not too severe, can open the door to creative expression. The child who uses artistic skill and self-determination to save himself or herself may find that artistic inclinations are closer to second nature than might otherwise be the case.

Does a psychological sensitivity manifest itself in my photographs? When I take a picture, I am reacting to the colors, the pat-

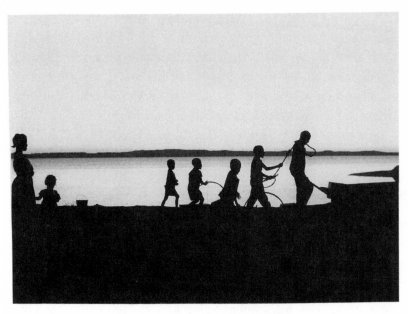

Barbara Young, *Twilight Parade*

terns, the feel. I don't think, "What does this mean?" But people examining my images have been reminded of certain associations, even in their dreams. In response to a photo entitled "Uffizi Landing" (plate 5), one observer wrote, "I wanted to *be* that little blue boat safely docked across all that water . . . safely moored to someone else. I didn't know if the larger boat felt like a parent or a partner . . . I just longed to be connected. . . . The feeling is enormously comforting."

My two careers seem to be intimately connected. In each I try to reestablish a state of equilibrium, to face conflict in order to resolve it. "The Creative Way of Life," a talk I have given often over the years, is an attempt to share with others my views on life and art. I encourage people to take time from their busy lives to get to know themselves. If they can tolerate the possible anxiety and "down" feeling elicited by looking inside the self, a resurgence of well-being, rejuvenation, and even inspiration will follow and perhaps set the hand to moving.

My creativity gives meaning to my life. It is the core of my existence; it is where my soul resides. As I grow older, death becomes more imminent. My circle of friends is rapidly diminishing. Will I be next? Was I self-indulgent in choosing to be an artist? My Puritan conscience twinges, though I know I could not have done otherwise. The creative push was too strong. I do not want to be like the man who said on his deathbed, "I've never done anything in my life that I most wanted to do!" It is better to have lived with a little guilt than with many regrets.

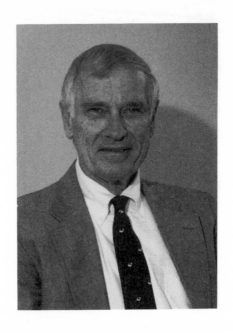

WAYNE O. SOUTHWICK is an orthopedic surgeon and sculptor, several of whose works adorn the grounds of the Yale–New Haven Medical Center. As a child, Southwick was fascinated by three-dimensional images, first in nature and then in sculpture and architecture. He describes how medicine, especially orthopedics, blends with sculpture in a visual and humane way. Dr. Southwick provides inspiration to other physicians, because only late in his career did he realize the talents that his work in orthopedics had helped shape. Now retired, he devotes all his time to sculpture.

From Bone to Stone

Wayne O. Southwick, M.D.

When I decided to take up sculpture at the age of fifty-six, my life was already too full: my medical practice was booming, my teaching and academic obligations were more than I could bear, and I was recovering from a fourth operation on my back. But I have always loved the three-dimensional quality of this art form: it has mass, occupies space, and can be seen from many angles. Size, material, surface, and color, along with space, lighting, and surroundings, all profoundly affect its appearance. Sculpture has texture; much of it is appreciated through touch as well as through sight. (Many great sculptures have been touched to such an extent that some of the stone, bronze, or other material has been worn away.) Touch, as one of the most primitive and important of our senses, often has a powerful effect on our perceptions.

Why I have been fascinated by sculpture is not clear. It may have been my early exposure to the barren landscapes of Friend, Nebraska, a community of eleven hundred people, mostly farmers who depended entirely on the land. The landscape comprised a relentlessly flat prairie, a big sky, and an ocean of wheat, corn, soybeans, and grass dotted with an occasional barn, windmill, silo, or grain elevator and, of course, cattle and horses. Aspects of this scene, such as the billowing white clouds that at dawn and dusk turned purple and orange, seemed largely two-dimensional. The spaciousness and flatness made human artifacts stand out as three-dimensional interruptions that could be felt as well as seen. Looking back, I think it was the impact of those large objects on the land that gave me an interest in sculpture.

In the mornings I would sometimes watch the steam trains scream by our little depot at ninety miles an hour as a trainman threw off the bundle of newspapers I was to deliver. Waiting beforehand on the tracks, I could see the wide straight rails narrow into the horizon eighteen miles away. I imagined I could see—and eventually I actually would see—a tiny speck on the track on the east horizon that grew larger as it approached. In the last quarter mile, a gigantic engine, freight cars, and a caboose would zoom by like a bolt of lightning, the noise of the whistle, the wind, and the clicking wheels almost deafening me. Then, in less than a minute, the vision would be gone. Often I watched until it passed the tall grain elevators in Exeter, the next little town, and again became a speck on the western horizon.

This massive intrusion changed the silent two-dimensional landscape into a palpable and audible three-dimensional extravaganza. We also played in and on all of these large objects. Although forbidden to do so by the railroad, we often climbed up the tall iron ladders to the top of the empty boxcars parked on the side tracks and jumped ten or fifteen feet into sandpiles alongside. These grand volumes—the barns, elevators, silos, windmills, and boxcars—so huge to us, were scarcely noticeable on the vast prairie. Perhaps they could be thought of as our sculptures.

I remember some other large objects. Among the statues on the Nebraska State Capitol building is *The Sower,* by Lee Laurie, a nineteen-foot bronze of a farmer casting grain from a sack. It sits atop the two-hundred-foot tower of the new capitol, visible for twenty miles across the wheat fields surrounding Lincoln. On the west lawn stands an elegant bronze of Abraham Lincoln by Daniel Chester French, along with a stone slab on which the Gettysburg Address is carved. In Morrill Hall on the University of Nebraska campus is a life-size copy of Venus. Although all these objects were fascinating, I had no thought at the time of attempting to sculpt myself.

In 1937, a cross-country train trip to Washington, D.C., for the first International Boy Scout Jamboree exposed me to remarkable art and architecture. In New York I saw Paul Manship's *Prometheus* at

Rockefeller Center and the Statue of Liberty in the harbor. In the District of Columbia, we camped on the Mall between the Washington Monument and the Lincoln Memorial. The many statues of generals on horseback in that city are some of my fondest memories.

By age fifteen I had begun to think about becoming a physician. Our family doctor, Rodney K. Johnson, also my scoutmaster, seemed enthusiastic about everything he did, even in the midst of the drought and the Depression; everyone in our little town admired him. I focused on medicine and chemistry because my brother was training to become an organic chemist. My favorite course in high school was solid geometry, probably because of its three-dimensional aspects. As valedictorian of my class, I won a regents' scholarship to the University of Nebraska.

Shortly before Pearl Harbor, I joined the navy's V-12 program for premedical students. We were required to complete the required courses and enter medical school in the shortest possible time. I took an optional drawing course but no sculpture. My most interesting undergraduate course was comparative zoology, which involved the dissection of frogs and cats. I now think that the three-dimensional forms of these animals, the individual muscles we dissected, their attachment to the bones, and their relationship to the nerves and blood vessels were similar to the disciplines of surgery and sculpture.

In May 1944, during my medical training, I married Ann Seacrest. Because of the complexities of our life—I was learning medicine, surgery, and orthopedics, going off to Korea as a naval medical officer, and working my way up through the ranks of academic medicine—she ended up raising our three children virtually alone. In the course of these years, we moved thirteen times.

Medical school was extremely intense and stressful; for example, about one-third of the entering class at the University of Nebraska was eliminated in the first year. Fortunately, Dr. John S. Latta, the chair of anatomy and the person deciding who remained and who did not, encouraged me and gave me a high ranking. Even though anatomy was difficult because I had to learn an entirely new vocabulary, I enjoyed performing the dissections, examining the structures, and understanding their three-dimensional relationships. During my clinical years he appointed me an assistant in anatomy and histology to help teach first-year students, mostly veterans returning from the war. Dr. Latta also helped to arrange my internship and residency training at Boston City Hospital, where Tufts has a medical program and Harvard a surgical service. Another of my jobs was taking electrocardiograms (EKGs) for the University of Nebraska Hospital. Ann had become an X-ray technician, so I became familiar with these two fields by being present as cardiologists and radiologists made their diagnoses. The EKGs of cardiology and the films of radiology are, in my opinion, like drawings. Other fields such as endocrinology or psychiatry involve mostly abstract reasoning and are neither visual nor palpable. This lack of perceptible form may be why I was always drawn to gross anatomy, histology, radiology, cardiology, and surgery —all strongly visual.

At Boston City Hospital I soon learned that the three-dimensional fields (such as surgery, neurosurgery, and orthopedics) fascinated me much more than two-dimensional realms (cardiology and radiology). While on the Harvard surgical service, I rotated to the Harvard neurological unit and the fracture service. As a result, I learned how broken bones could be restored to their correct anatomical position, mostly by touch. If one could feel beneath the skin, find where the muscles were to be inserted, and then apply appropriate forces to bring them back into position, restoration was often simple and dramatic. By palpation, by knowing the correct location of muscle and bony landmarks, one could carefully wrap a plaster cast and hold the bone fragments in their proper location until the cast set. I also learned how to repair fractured hips, which required an exact understanding of the location of the femoral head, without exposing it surgically—another important three-dimensional problem.

Although I enjoyed general surgery and the surgical specialties, they did not contain all the elements of form and function, as orthopedics did. I could have remained in general surgery or neurosurgery, but I chose to go into orthopedics at Johns Hopkins Hospital.

During my house-staff years in Boston, looking at sculpture had become a growing pleasure; Ann and I frequented the Museum of Fine Arts, a diversion we could afford. While Ann was viewing the Chagalls, the Impressionists, and the Picassos, I was studying the excellent collection of ancient Greek and Roman sculptures.

On my first visit to Baltimore, I entered Johns Hopkins Hospital via the Broadway entrance, with its vast dome and stairway and the statue of Christ by Thoraldson in the center of the rotunda. I was emotionally hooked. This became an architectural and sculptural holy space; from that moment on, I wanted to be a part of Johns Hopkins medicine. The impressive hill on which the building is situated, the circular brick driveway, the steps, and the entrance doors into the domed room bring to mind those great nineteenth-century individuals who planned and created this institution. As a house officer (an apt title for the trainees who lived and worked in the hospital in the sense that one was always "in the house"), my room was at the top of the five flights of stairs, just under the dome. I was usually so exhausted that I could barely make it to the top to crawl into bed, where I would collapse into unconsciousness. In spite of exhaustion, any lover of sculpture could not fail to feel the beauty and grandeur of this space under the dome.

I was privileged to be at Johns Hopkins Hospital from 1950 to 1958, except for my time as a navy medical officer at Bethesda and in Korea. Under Dr. Robert A. Robinson, we house officers became much more aware of the posture, anatomy, symmetry, and form of the body—especially the spine. We studied normal and abnormal kinematics, scoliosis, and limb deformities and their management, all of which required a strong three-dimensional understanding of the human form and the ability to feel the skeletal, muscular, and ligamentous landmarks and to understand how they related to one another. Once I had become an assistant professor and Dr. Robinson's only full-time assistant, I never thought of leaving that hospital. His creative energy, his love for his patients, his ability to detect through his fingers and vision the slightest deviations from the normal form, and his clinical depth and surgical skills spilled over onto those who worked under him.

By this time Ann and I had rented a tiny colonial farmhouse on a six-hundred-acre estate on the outskirts of the city. We nonetheless made frequent cultural forays to the Baltimore Museum of Art, which had a rich sculpture collection, including many pieces by Aristide Maillol.

When Dr. Gustav Lindskog, chair of the Department of Surgery at Yale, offered me the position of chief of orthopedics there, none of the family wanted to leave Baltimore. And because I was only thirty-five, I couldn't believe the offer was serious. Dr. Lindskog phoned when I had not responded and asked me to visit New Haven. After showing me around for the better part of a day, he requested that I write down what was needed to make orthopedics a strong section at Yale. Although I wanted to stay at Hopkins, Robinson thought I should take the position at Yale and helped me compile a list. So the family left Baltimore in July 1958, everyone in tears as the old station wagon pulled away. I have been at Yale ever since.

Moving back into a city was a shock for all of us, but we finally adapted. We often went to the Yale Art Gallery and to the Metropolitan Museum and the Museum of Modern Art in New York. Maillol's peaceful, classical, and geometric style became my favorite, and I found myself returning over and over to study his sculptures.

Ann and I had never considered buying any original artwork—until a trip to Paris in 1959. There Ann purchased several signed Chagall prints at the Louvre for less than one hundred dollars, which turned out to be a marvelous investment. I spent my time in the Louvre looking at the *Winged Victory,* the *Venus de Milo,* and the Maillols. Back home, as a member of a committee that met in Chicago, I tried to spend time in the Chicago Art Institute, which was only a block from the meetings. In the museum shop I bought a little Maillol statuette of bronzed plaster, which I kept on my desk. Not until 1965 did I consider trying to make sculpture myself. That year I volunteered for two months on the medical ship *Hope,* which was headed to the impoverished country of Guinea, West Africa, to offer free medical care to the natives. On the way home I arranged to take two days in Paris to visit the museums and the Dina Vernay Gallery, which sold Maillol sculptures. I saw a beautiful statuette for eighteen hundred dollars, but I felt we couldn't afford it. At that point I began to think I should try to make something like it myself. (In 1996, at a Maillol exhibit in New York City, a similar statuette was selling for thirty thousand dollars.)

I did not actually try to sculpt until 1977. We were invited to the home of Adlai Hardin, a retired businessman who had taken up sculpture at age fifty-five. I admired his fine wood carvings, mostly of religious figures such as Adam and Eve, Saint Paul, and Saint Peter, as well as some lovely torsos and portraits in bronze. As he showed me his studio, I asked him if he would consider giving me lessons. He seemed interested, but we failed to get together. One fall, after he and his family had returned from vacation in northern Wisconsin, his wife called and asked if I would request a lesson. On vacation he had suddenly lost the sight of his right eye and had not returned to his studio; she thought I might get him started again. At first he hesitated when I asked, but finally he agreed to meet me at his studio the next day. We started by each making a clay torso from a picture in one of Maillol's books.

After finishing the clays, we made molds. Mine he converted to plaster; his became a beautiful wood carving, which he sold for a sizable fee. From there he went on to fill many commissions, including the large sculptures of Saint Peter and Saint Paul that adorn the entrance to Saint Patrick's Cathedral on Fifth Avenue in New York.

After our sessions, Adlai suggested that I take some lessons at a new local art school, the Lyme Academy of Fine Arts. I declined because of lack of time. In 1979, however, I took a leave of absence from the medical school to recover from my fourth spinal operation. I rested for a month, then enrolled in drawing under Dean Keller and in sculpture under Michael Lantz and Elisabeth Gordon Chandler (the founder of the school). All three are superb artists and teachers and gave me an excellent start. With continuing instruction from the academy, especially from Dean Keller, Laci de Gerenday, and Don Gale, I have since spent one day a week working at sculpture.

In 1985 I began to take special classes with Bruno Lucchesi, an internationally known sculptor who works primarily in terra-cotta and bronze. It has been my good fortune to be around this fine sculptor for the past few years. His work, best seen in published volumes, rivals that of renowned Renaissance artists—Donatello, Michelangelo, Canova, Verrocchio, and others. Unfortunately, there seem to be no modern popes or world bankers to act as patrons for Lucchesi's magnificent larger-than-life sculptures.

The first opportunity to display my work occurred in 1992, when Dr. Peter Jokl, director of Yale Sports Medicine Center, asked me to create a life-size sculpture for the building's fifteen-foot atrium.

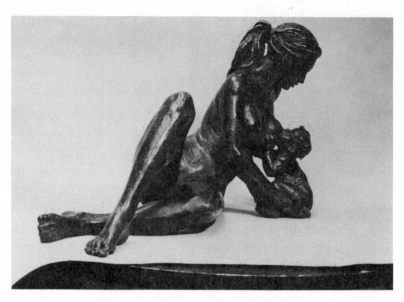

Wayne Southwick, *Taking Nourishment*

The result is a ten-foot bronze named *An American Dream* (plate 6). In approaching this commission, I began to think about how sports had produced more integration of minorities than any other activity and about what it was doing to realize the dream of Martin Luther King, Jr.: that one day his children would be judged more by the quality of their deeds and their spirit than by the color of their skin. Also, I wanted to acknowledge that women are becoming better recognized in sports and are often winning over men these days. I hoped to portray not only the action of sport but its spiritual and physical beauty as well. One day while reading the *Friend (Nebraska) Sentinel,* my hometown paper, I spotted photographs of the girls' basketball team of Friend High School, which had won the regional tournament. Photos of those teenagers leaping high in the air triggered my idea of a woman jumping to shoot a basket while a male player watched.

Another sculpture, entitled *Taking Nourishment,* depicts a two-year-old baby nursing from his mother in a pose reminiscent of the famous bronze of Romulus and Remus nursing from the she-wolf. This piece is intended to remind one that as the young become older and stronger, they often take more and more from their mothers (and fathers).

Although teaching and academic orthopedics continually presented me with new and interesting challenges, my encounter with sculpture has provided endless opportunities to explore new ideas and new ways of expressing artistically the human spirit, form, and fantasy. Great sculptures seem almost alive; one can sense their beauty and rhythm. The creation of a sculpture of value is elusive, but enormous satisfaction results if others seem to enjoy your work.

A fascinating world has been opened to me through a series of somewhat random events. I am incredibly lucky to have received so much from so many wonderful teachers, residents, and students. Surprisingly, the sculpture of the basketball players at the medical school made me better known as a sculptor than as a teacher or surgeon. Probably not many of us in academic medicine have been so fortunate.

Part 2

Music

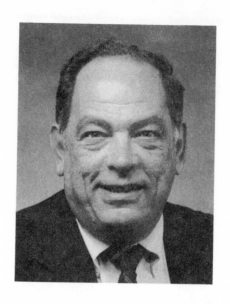

A gastroenterologist and jazz musician, J A M E S C E R D A learned to play the piano at the age of three and was soon composing. A longtime interest in the navy interrupted his intention of becoming a composer and concert pianist and led to his enlistment during the Korean War. After four years of active duty, he remained in the Naval Reserve, retiring in 1990 as a rear admiral, possibly the only gastroenterologist to enjoy that title as more than a joke. Now a professor of medicine at the University of Florida, Cerda shares with us his fascination with some famous musician-physicians, fitting them into the mosaic of his own life. Cerda continues to play and compose music and has joined a number of jazz bands whose concerts benefit charity.

In the Key of Sea

James J. Cerda, M.D.

Western medicine has always focused on the mechanistic aspects of illness and health, with scant regard to human beings as whole systems. But the solution to many medical problems may not lie in the realm of chemical, pharmacological, or even physical therapies. By contrast, the Chinese approach to medicine has always emphasized the mind-body connection, including the influence of the arts. Scholars of the Han dynasty, for example, recognized that music affected the body physiologically by calming the spirit and stimulating circulation.

Arts medicine is increasingly being recognized as an important synthesis, one that explores the impact of aesthetic stimuli (color, form, rhythm, sound) on human physiology; the neurophysiologic nature of creativity; the effect of the arts on early brain development; and their role in breaking down language and cultural barriers, humanizing modern medical institutions, and creating individual and cultural well-being.

I have always been fascinated, in particular, by the association between music and medicine and by the many well-known musicians who were also trained as physicians —Fritz Kreisler, Hermann Boerhaave, Hector Berlioz, Theodor Billroth, and Albert Schweitzer, to name a few.

The child prodigy Fritz Kreisler, born in Vienna in 1875, won the Grand Prix of the Paris Conservatory at age twelve and the Prix de Rome at twenty. After a successful tour of the United States as a concert violinist, he gave up music for the study of medicine and was appointed a medical officer in the Austrian army. Music was his first love, however, and he soon abandoned medicine to become a celebrated violin virtuoso. In 1935 he confessed that a number of compositions that he had performed as "compositions of old masters" were, in fact, his own.

Hermann Boerhaave, born in 1668, was educated with the hope that he would follow in the footsteps of his cleric father. The greatest clinician and medical educator of his time and a gifted linguist, Boerhaave was truly a Renaissance man. Less well known is that he developed the botanical garden in Leyden and was the first physician to fund the performance of chamber music.

Berlioz was the son of a small-town physician who had little sympathy for his son's musical career. His father, Louis, exerted every possible influence to direct Hector into medicine, the choice of Hector's grandfather and uncle as well. Fortunately for music, Bernard Vandiern, a great composer, quickly recognized Hector as a child prodigy and gifted musician. He stated that "with the sole exception of Mozart," Berlioz possessed "the most stupendous gifts of the past century."

Nevertheless, Berlioz entered medical school and graduated in 1824. His desire to be a musician, however, proved stronger than his conscription into the medical profession. Against the advice of friends and his parents (who threatened to cut off his allowance), he attended classes given by the noted composer Jean-François Lesueur. After hearing Berlioz's mass, the master stated, "You should not be a doctor or a druggist, or anything else, but a great musician." Stubbornly, his father held that Hector should continue with medicine and did allow him to pursue his musical ambitions. Berlioz's lifestyle, marked by unsuccessful love affairs and a lack of money, was an impediment. Niccolò Paganini also recognized Berlioz's phenomenal ability and after a performance of *Harold* in Italy paid tribute to him by getting down on his knees and congratulating him. It was through Paganini and Baron de Rothschild that Berlioz was able to complete *Romeo and Juliet* and his magnificent *Symphonie fantastique,* works that established him as an outstanding composer. (Incidentally, Paganini may have suffered from Marfan's syndrome, which in conferring him with long fingers and hyperextensive joints probably contributed to his manual dexterity and his reputation as the greatest violin virtuoso of all time.)

Although Theodor Billroth's pioneering surgery of the digestive tract gained him international recognition, his true ambitions lay in music. Nevertheless, his parents opposed his early hope to study music and insisted on a career in medicine. Billroth met Johannes Brahms in Zurich, and the two formed a lifelong friendship. The leading musicians of Vienna gathered at Billroth's home for evenings of music, with Billroth performing on piano or violin; virtually all of Brahms's chamber music was played there for the first time. Billroth also wrote extensively, and in *Wer Ist Musicalisch?* he attempted to develop a physiologic theory of music appreciation. He was recognized as a music critic and wrote reviews for the magazine *Neue Zürcher Zeitung*.

Albert Schweitzer developed a love of music early in his life, as a pupil of Eugene Munch, one of Germany's most illustrious organists. Under Munch's tutelage, Schweitzer developed as a great organist and an outstanding interpreter of Bach. In 1893, Schweitzer entered the University of Strasbourg, where he studied philosophy, theology, and music. In 1900 he was ordained a Lutheran minister and began to write extensively on theology. Five years later, a published plea by the president of a Paris missionary society for volunteers to work in Africa led Schweitzer to serve as a medical missionary. Again he enrolled in the University of Strasbourg, this time to prepare himself to work as a physician in French Equatorial Africa. His legendary work there led to his winning the Nobel Prize. Despite failing health, he continued to give lectures and concerts in many European countries, using the proceeds to fund hospitals in Africa.

My love of music developed early. Under the tutelage of my mother, who had studied and taught piano before her marriage, I began playing at age three; by seven I was composing. My principal instructor was Glenn Carow, an internationally known pianist who included some of my compositions in his performances at Constitution Hall in Washington, D.C.

In 1949–50, I was taking courses at George Washington University, the Catholic School of Music, and the Peabody Conservatory, with the thought of a career on the concert stage. But the Korean War came along and changed all that. Rather than be drafted into the army, I chose to enlist in the navy, which had held an appeal for me even as a child. During my interview with a navy recruiter, I stated that I was a concert pianist. "Good," he responded, "you'll make a great typist." I was sent to personnel school, where I learned to type more than one hundred words per minute!

Four years of active duty did not deter me from my musical pursuits. During my several tours of duty with the Sixth Fleet, I played for numerous radio programs, under the sponsorship of the Voice of America, and appeared as a soloist at the Venice Art Festival. These experiences, however, convinced me that a career as a concert pianist was not to be. Medicine immediately seemed a natural alternative in that I had always done well in science and was strongly attracted to the idea of doing medical research. In 1957 I entered the University of Maryland School of Medicine.

Even during medical school, I continued to play and to compose. Some of my most memorable performances include those for presidents Truman, Eisenhower, and Kennedy, the latter when I was a medical resident. In addition, I played with the Paul Whiteman Orchestra, broadcast my own radio program on WGAY in Washington, D.C., and appeared on numerous television shows.

During the 1940s I had also developed a strong interest in jazz. In 1948 I met Jim Parker, now Dr. James Parker, an eminent psychologist in the Washington area. We were both intrigued by modern jazz, particularly the complex music known as bebop. The two of us played in clubs in the Washington area, with a number of musicians who went on to stardom.

In 1972 I moved to Gainesville to join the faculty of the University of Florida College of Medicine. There I joined an eighteen-piece big band that played mainly the Count Basie book. We began to give concerts to raise money for the Hazel Donegan Medical Scholarship Fund. In addition, for the past fifteen years or so I have played in a group known as "The Docs of Dixieland." The original "Docs" included Dr. Charles Cusumano (trumpet), an oncologist; Dr. Hal Bingham (clarinet), a plastic surgeon; and Dr. Rod Millian (drums), a radiation oncologist. Over the years, several dozen "Docs" played with the group, depending on who was in town. Medical stu-

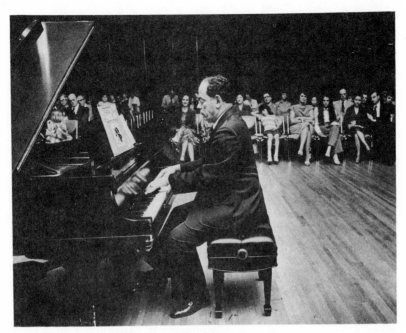
James Cerda performing at a benefit concert

dents and physicians have come and gone, owing to the demands of academic medicine. Nor have all members been physicians (a banker, a business executive, a music professor, and a restaurateur have sat in with us), though as the leader of the group I feel authorized to "bless" them as "Docs." Having completely funded the Hazel Donegan Fund, we are now working on a scholarship for the Department of Music. In addition, I have given numerous benefit performances, including a recent solo concert for the Multiple Sclerosis Society.

Throughout this time, however, I could never get the navy out of my system. I joined the Naval Reserve as a third-year medical student and retired in 1990 as a rear admiral. Again, music remained an integral part of the experiece: I was always asked to play at meetings of my fellow flag officers.

Music is an art to which many physicians are attracted, whether as performers or as listeners. The reason for this affinity will continue to fuel speculation, all the more as therapeutic goals are pursued through interdisciplinary research involving physiology, psychology, music, and medicine. Neuroscientists are currently interested, for example, in locating the area of musical talent in the brain.

At the University of Florida, we have established an Art in Medicine group. Its purpose is to encourage caring and humanistic communication among health professionals and patients through art and music and to provide artists a new dimension in which to express their art as an integral part of the healing process. The goals of this cooperative effort are fivefold: to improve humanistic communication between doctor and patient and among health professionals; to encourage artistic expression among health professionals by bringing to their attention international figures who have combined science and art; to create an awareness of the symbiotic relationship of the arts and human physiology in the healing process and the prevention of illness, with special reference to such new areas of scientific exploration as psychoneuroimmunology; to form a dedicated group of artists and scientists willing to interact with patients suffering from terminal or chronic illness in an attempt to encourage the expression of their pain, fears, and hopes and to improve the quality of their lives through some form of art or art appreciation; and to collect data relative to the response of patients, artists, and health professionals involved in the program.

The creative arts reawaken the awareness of the original Hippocratic principles upon which medicine was founded, principles that focus on humanism, harmony, and quality of life rather than on the unattainable goal of curing all known disease. Art opens us to our humanness, helping us to communicate with, enlighten, and inspire others. The complementary aspects of art and science relate directly to the wellness-illness dichotomy. The best art and the best medical science breathe new life into the human experience.

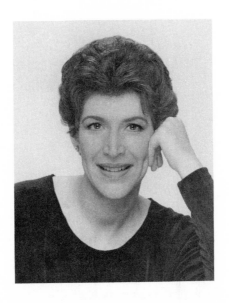

An endocrinologist at New York's Mount Sinai
Hospital during the day and a cabaret singer at night,
ALICE LEVINE has successfully combined her
two aspirations. Medicine and singing have so fulfilled
her life that she cannot conceive of one without the
other: both are about communication with others and
both require creativity, discipline, and attention to
details. Good teachers are always on stage, so learning
to perform well in any field enhances their skills. Dr.
Levine is delighted that much of her audience is drawn
from health-care professionals, because, as she wryly
notes, "they certainly need some entertainment!"

The Singing Endocrinologist

Alice Levine, M.D.

T ruth be told, I never dreamt of becoming a doctor. As a child growing up in Brooklyn in the 1950s and 1960s, I imagined myself a famous singer. I enjoyed music from an early age and sang for the sheer joy of it. On cold days, I would wrap a scarf around my face and sing songs to pass the time as I walked to and from school.

I began college at the State University of New York at Albany in September 1970. During my first year, I remember attending teas in various departments in an effort to choose my major. Thoughts of a premed major were dampened by doubts about my scientific abilities. Although my mother was a professional (a clinical psychologist), it seemed more likely to me that I would marry a doctor than become one. The teas and cookies were excellent in the French department, and I had an ear for languages and a love of literature, so I became a French major.

Upon graduation from college, I moved to Manhattan to try to make it as a singer. It soon became apparent that I would need a steady source of income while awaiting my big break. That turned out to be a job at Mount Sinai Hospital in the Department of Neoplastic Diseases. I do not remember my exact job description—it was something like clinical research records coordinator—but I clearly remember my first day there. The chief of the department put a white coat on me and led me on rounds to see the cancer patients. I was frightened and overwhelmed by what I saw, but also excited by the experience. The next two years I worked closely with a female physician, and given this new role model, I began to entertain the possibility of becoming a physician myself. My increasing interest in medicine led me back to school; at Columbia University, I completed premed courses at the School of General Studies and continued my studies at the College of Physicians and Surgeons.

Between my college years and my entry into medical school in 1977, I had seen a bit of the world of show business, having appeared in summer stock and a few productions in New York. There were so many gifted performers out there looking for work, but I had begun to understand that talent was not enough. It was discouraging to think that one could be talented, work hard, take lessons, do everything the right way, and still not find a job in ten years' time. Success in show business seemed out of my control and dependent upon the fashion of the day and the whims of agents, directors, and audiences. To paraphrase Shakespeare, building a career in music was like climbing steps of sand.

Medicine is different. I think of the profession not only as a career but as a trade. I have a skill that does not depend upon any current trend, that goes with me wherever I go. Even with recent and future changes in the field, I feel empowered by the training and expertise I acquired during medical school. At Columbia, I found many other students who had come to medicine from diverse fields. My freshman year I starred in a medical school production (presented by the Bard Hall Players) of "Wonderful Town," and I joined a band named "Arrhythmia," led by my talented classmate Robert Golub. During my first two years of medical school, I actually had quite a lot of show business experience; these diversions in fact made my studies easier, not more difficult.

After graduation, I completed an internal medicine residency and then returned to Mount Sinai Medical Center for a fellowship in endocrinology, a field I chose for many reasons. I have always preferred having time to think about problems, and I enjoy knowing that most endocrine puzzles can be solved and that most patients can be treated. I find it fascinating that estradiol and testosterone are so chemically similar yet have such opposite effects in the human body. During my fellowships I began a research project on hormonal treatment of benign prostatic hyperplasia. Through that project, I met my husband, an academic urologist. We are presently codirectors of a basic research laboratory investigating the interaction of sex steroids and growth factors in the human prostate.

In spite of the new challenges in my life, I began to miss my music. One evening while flipping through cable television, I came across my former mentor in cabaret, John Wallowitch, performing piano requests on a phone-in show. At that moment I decided to create a cabaret show of my own. I knew that, realistically, I could not audition for shows or movies and continue to have a medical career. Cabaret is the only art form in which the performer has complete control. Needless to say, putting together a cabaret show involves the investment of time, work, and money. On the other hand, it is a creative and rewarding experience and can be undertaken in off-hours.

Prior to medical school, I had been working with John but had never managed to actually perform cabaret. After medical school and residency, I had a new perspective, in that neither my livelihood nor my sense of self-esteem depended on the show. In short, I was much more confident and willing to take chances. As I said in one of my shows, being a doctor totally changed my approach to auditions. I would think to myself: "Well, what is the worst that can happen on this audition? Maybe the director or producer won't like me or won't give me the job, but at least no one is going to get sick and die during the audition."

I now try to put together a cabaret show once a year. Most recently, I performed at two clubs on West Forty-sixth Street in Manhattan, Danny's Skylight Room and Don't Tell Mama. I enjoy the process of choosing material and creating an entertaining performance. My song selection is, to say the least, eclectic. I choose songs that elicit strong reactions when I first hear them—either laughter or tears. John Wallowitch is a wonderful songwriter, as able with ballads as he is with funny material, and I generally include several of his songs (among them "Come a Little Closer," "After All," and the outrageous "Bruce," about a cross-dresser with terrible taste in clothing). Poring over his considerable collection of old songs often provides me with some beauties ("April in Fairbanks," by Murray Grand; "Rhode Island Is Famous for You," by Dietz and Schwartz). On a light note, I enjoy finding mock audition numbers that I might have done for stage or movie parts (for example, a Sheldon Harnick song named "Garbage," done with a Spanish accent). Out of nostalgia for my roots, I sometimes perform an old song by Dan Shapiro, Milton Pascal, and Phil Charig entitled "I'm Gonna Hang My Hat on a Tree That Grows in Brooklyn." When it comes to ballads, I rely on Wallowitch tunes, the old standards, and quite a few Billy Joel songs ("Leningrad," "And So It Goes"). I'm happy to say that my shows have been well received by critics, family, and friends.

The two careers are, in many ways, very similar. Both singing and medicine are about communicating with people, and both require not only creativity but tremendous discipline and attention to details. As faculty at an academic medical center, I am required to do a lot of teaching. My cabaret days have enhanced these skills immensely, for I know that to get a message across I must be not only informative but also clear, direct, and entertaining.

Conversely, my experiences as a physician have influenced my cabaret selections. Although I still enjoy singing a heart-wrenching ballad, I try to juxtapose serious moments with lighter ones. Much of my audience is made up of my colleagues in the health-care profession —and they certainly need some entertainment!

When I first returned to cabaret as a singing endocrinologist, I tried to keep these two worlds separate. Initially, I did not tell the medical world about my singing career, and in my first cabaret shows I never spoke of being a doctor. As I gained more experience, however, the two worlds began to interconnect. The news of my other career leaked out to my division chief, who promptly made a reservation to check out the situation. He loved the show, has returned time and time again, and even recruited me to perform at the annual fundraiser for Mount Sinai. When the chief of medicine saw the show, he came up with the idea of having all the faculty develop other careers in this era of managed care.

At first I felt that my patients and colleagues would not take me seriously as a doctor if they saw the show, but quite the opposite has occurred. Cabaret performances are intimate, and performers reveal a lot about themselves in those moments before the audience. Both patients and colleagues appreciate that sense of intimacy and seem to relate to me on a warmer, more personal basis afterward. I am still reluctant to tell my patients directly about my singing. My husband, however, is proud of my efforts and does not hesitate to tell his patients, many of whom see my shows.

During my first year in college, when I was searching for some concrete meaning in my education, my mother advised me that a liberal arts education would probably prepare me more for my life from five to nine than from nine to five. As I grow older, I realize that different aspects of a person's existence cannot be compartmentalized. That realization has made me more comfortable with the fusion of my two careers into one rewarding life.

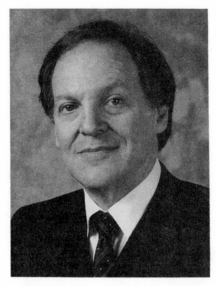

Todd Geig

As a music major at Yale, ELI NEWBERGER

played the tuba with the New Haven Symphony. Since

graduating from medical school, he has enjoyed music

as a second career. To satisfy his sense of adventure, he

joined the Peace Corps and was sent to Africa, where he

learned more about the origins of jazz. Africa not only

nurtured his interest in child health and development

but also convinced him that music could be a life's

calling. As medical director of the Family Development

Program at Children's Hospital in Boston, he daily faces

the daunting problems of child abuse. The demands

of his medical life, however, are counterbalanced by

the emotional release he finds in his weekly gigs as a

tuba player in a jazz band.

Medicine of the Tuba

Eli Newberger, M.D.

I backed into medicine as an undergraduate at Yale. If I'd continued as a tuba player beyond the New Haven Symphony, I'd have ended up counting rests in an orchestra brass section. I never intended to leave music, but I could never have anticipated how my music major, and especially a music theory project on the evolution of jazz piano, would come to influence my choice of specialty and drive my medical career.

My transition from music to medical school in fall 1962 was eased by marriage to Carolyn Moore and by our summer work as aides in the children's program of the Connecticut Valley Hospital. At the end of my first year at Yale medical school, the joint position of resident directors of the International House became open. The opportunity to help foreign graduate students adjust to the rigors of life in New Haven in return for a free apartment was irresistible. In our three years there, my wife and I enjoyed the company of these sophisticated individuals, who hardly needed our guidance. At the same time she and I developed a lively antipathy to the war in Vietnam.

In 1966, when I graduated from medical school, all male medical graduates were subject to the draft. The most palatable alternative to the military was the U.S. Public Health Service, specifically the Peace Corps. Feeling adventurous, and fascinated by the origins of jazz, I put in for a post in Africa. In 1967 Carolyn and I left for Ouagadougou, Upper Volta (now Burkina Faso), with our five-week-old daughter.

My assignment was to provide medical care for the volunteers—forty-two healthy young Americans—and technical support for a weakly conceived maternal- and child-health program. The aim was to have raw college graduates teach African mothers how to make better use of locally available foodstuffs to prevent protein malnutrition and reduce infectious disease. The general medical job turned out to be a piece of cake; the latter, however, was a Peace Corps folly that contradicted deep traditions regarding the role of women and the care and feeding of infants. On the other hand, my rounding at Ouagadougou Hospital with Ezra Elian, an eminent Israeli pediatric professor sent as part of an aid program, led me to apply for a pediatric residency, which I would begin on completion of my two years in Africa.

Africa also convinced me that jazz would be another, equally important calling in my life. I occasionally played with a high-life band called Volta Jazz, made up of Upper Voltans from the city of Bobo Dioulasso. The rich, complex rhythms I discovered as part of this group were inspiring. I also struggled to learn the balafon, the African progenitor of the marimba. Shortly before our departure, I received a clipping from the *New Haven Register,* naming me as the originator of the jazz band at the International House, begun four years earlier in an effort to liven up our Friday night coffeehouse. The group, originally called the International Feetwarmers, was by then known as the Galvanized Washboard Band and was holding forth with a guest clarinetist from Harvard, Tommy Sancton. On moving to Boston in June 1969, I called Tommy, and with a British computer engineer, Tony Pringle, we started the Black Eagle Jazz Band, with Roy Smith on drums, Jim Klippert on trombone, Dave Duquette on banjo, and me on piano. When I switched to the tuba in 1971, we added "New" to the name. In the decades since then, we've played around the world; in 1996 we completed two European tours; our recordings, which now number about forty, continue to sell, if mostly to jazz cognoscenti.

We manage about one hundred gigs a year. The joy and release of this musical life has enabled me to deal with the rigors of child abuse and family violence: my medical life connects to the sense of shared struggle and social protest that runs deep in the history and practice of jazz. Without music, I could not have pursued this specialty within pediatrics, for reasons having to do with creative inspiration and the dampening of it; the opposing emotional tug of joy and despair; and the clarity that music brings to the personal and professional ambiguities of medical work.

I consider myself as much musician as physician. My life has been a constant balancing act, music sometimes serving as the counterweight to medicine, and sometimes the reverse.

In 1971 I was one year short of completing my pediatric training at Children's Hospital in Boston. A newly opened pub in Hopkinton, Massachusetts, hired our band for a trial one Sunday afternoon. The place sold out, and before long we were playing every Thursday night—in that Thursdays did not interfere with the weekend gigs that are a working musician's bread and butter. Soon we had a regular following and audience members from around the world.

That same year I was also taking a course at the Harvard School of Public Health, which required students to write a mock grant proposal. I proposed an investigation that would reclassify the problem of child abuse among the social illnesses of childhood. I suggested a new theory to explain abuse, failure to thrive, accidents, and poisonings in preschoolers: that underlying these "diseases" was a common causal matrix of social, family, and child-centered stresses, with varying combinations driving the expression of particular patterns.

We published an evaluation of how interdisciplinary coordination and case review reduced the monetary and human costs of child abuse and established one of the first outpatient clinics for abused and neglected children in the United States. We saw patients on Thursdays, because that was when space was available.

So ever since 1972, my Thursdays have been entirely committed. In the morning, I usually consult on the management of one or two abused or neglected children on the inpatient floors, talking with doctors, nurses, and social workers about their findings. Does the evidence merit making a required report to the state child-protection agency? Should a legal action on behalf of the child be filed in the juvenile court? Are other siblings, and the children's mother, also at risk of abuse? Or is it safe to send the child home?

Each year our hospital deals with five hundred cases of suspected child abuse or neglect, up from sixty-two in 1970. And the cases are complex, over half involving a mother who is also a victim of domestic violence. Defining how to help, without harming, is an ambiguous and confusing process. Fortunately, I work with committed, supportive colleagues in a hospital that has embraced the program.

On Thursday afternoons, until five o'clock, we see children, parents, grandparents, and stepparents. "See" is perhaps an understatement: interview, examine, and evaluate are more accurate. But even more apt descriptions of our interactions would be "share the pain" and "deal with the terror and trauma" of the children and women, which involves heartrending conflicts over a child's custody in the face of frightening allegations, few of which turn out to be false.

For all our professionalism, we cannot avoid getting drawn into family dramas. Inevitably, our findings displease someone, and we are subpoenaed to appear in court and subjected to the usual crossfire, during which our professed expertise is held up to ridicule. It is always chastening to be abused for trying to protect the abused. The work is not for the faint of heart. If we conclude, for example, that a four-year-old girl has been sexually abused by her mother's brother, the judge will sometimes indicate in his rulings that he doesn't believe such things actually happen.

As chief of the clinic, I observe and supervise interviews through a one-way mirror. From the darkened observation room, my colleagues and I often feel that we are peering into the worst miseries of people's lives. Few of us can imagine what it is like to be terrorized every day, to endure painful and humiliating assaults, and not to be believed. Of course I try my best to support my colleagues, who are also deeply affected by what they hear. As five o'clock draws near, it often seems as if we've all been through the wringer: eyes glisten, jaws clench, we slump in our chairs.

At five, I leave the clinic, and forty-five minutes later I pull into the parking lot outside Coffee, Tea, and Melody, the pub the Black Eagles have been playing since 1995. I take off my tie, pull the tuba out of the trunk, and enter a different world. Here, injustice does not prevail, there is sadness but not misery, and every moment of improvisation carries with it a prospect of redemption. Indeed, "mistakes" in jazz improvisation become platforms for new ideas, not catastrophes that destroy lives.

Inside Tony's already warming up his cornet with the simple blues lines he loves, and the room is filling with jazz fans, at least half of whom I know. Some members of the audience have been following the band for more than two decades; they feel like family. After a few greetings, I take my seat on a bar stool and begin to warm up with an arpeggio or two. Stan Vincent, the trombone player, arrives and gets ready to play. Then Tony plays the little bugle call that for twenty-nine years has been the signal for everyone to get ready. Tony greets the crowd and calls the first tune (usually something straightforward like "When I Grow Too Old to Dream" or "Moose March"; it's comfortable to begin with a nice New Orleans tune, though the band has a repertoire of some seven hundred numbers). Stan looks quizzical and asks what key it's in. The crowd laughs, because they've seen this act before, but Tony tells him anyway that it's in F and kicks off the tune by stamping his heel.

At this point my life is completely transformed. As we begin our first tune, everything else flows out of my mind. The ensemble is rich, thick, warm, and lively, with seven distinctive, familiar voices. I am always surprised by how wonderful it sounds. The beat is propulsive and swinging; and the tuba in my arms actually disappears from my consciousness.

From some place within me comes a series of notes, not exactly a tune, but a low melodic line that both buttresses the ensemble and propels the rhythm. I "think" the notes—that is, I imagine a set of sounds—and they simply emerge from the horn. As I do this, I feel I am reaching the people in the audience, both their ears and their hearts.

This is not, strictly speaking, a conscious process. As I play, I do not focus on what I am doing with the tuba to produce the sounds; it all happens spontaneously, and quickly. (If you stopped me and asked me at any moment, though, I could tell you exactly what I was doing and exactly what note each member of the band was playing.) In the middle of making music, I'm thinking colors, textures, and feelings, not notes and chords.

As the tune moves along, Tony distributes solos, mostly by his sense of who can best contribute as the piece evolves, sometimes in keeping with how the tune was treated by an artist or composer in the 1920s or 1930s. We pay homage to our musical forebears but avoid recapitulating note for note the original versions. The task in traditional jazz is to make the tradition come alive.

Sometimes, the day's events will impinge on my thoughts. This can actually displace the music to what I think of as another register in my mind. I'll weigh the thought in question and go on automatic pilot, tracing the bass line of the song. If Tony calls me to solo, I'll instantly forget whatever was distracting me, walk forward with the tuba and, as we say, take my chorus. In jazz, this means making up your own melody over the underlying chords, for twelve, sixteen, or thirty-two measures. In traditional or New Orleans–style jazz, there are strict improvisational rules; one works within them to make an emotionally honest, interesting, and original statement.

Inevitably, you make mistakes—that is, you play notes that do not belong in the harmony. But you always recover, and even profit, from such moments, which add excitement and chance to the unfolding expression of musical ideas. This is what I mean in referring to the promise of redemption. The improvisation is a kind of subversive play. One deliberately contorts the melody, creating something different and personal. A good chorus is intellectually engaging, a statement of the player's view of the world. The solo should also resonate to the underlying feel of the tune. Not a few songs evoke the hardships and travails of the human experience, as well as the shared aspiration for overcoming them. Jazz is a music of protest and possibility. For me, it offers succor and relief from the oppressive aspects of my medical work. Without it, I might well become inured, hardened, and less able to feel for my patients and their families.

Our music elicits feelings that obviously relate to life experiences: joy, sadness, pride, love, lust, which are sometimes further evoked by the lyrics of a song. A happy tune, such as "Spreading Joy" or "Bogalusa Strut" can go far toward curing the blues. Some emotions, however, are almost impossible to name, and these can be expressed in strange convergences: the music can summon rage, shame, isolation, tenderness, aching, and painful contemplation of beauty.

I sense that my feelings are also felt by others, by band members as well as the audience. Mostly I play with my eyes closed, but sometimes when my feelings almost overwhelm me, I'll open my eyes. Then I see that what I'm feeling is real. Before me are tears, rapt expressions, faces full of love. It's not by chance that some of the best jazz recordings are the product of live settings, as opposed to a recording studio. Contact with the audience is vital to this music.

I should mention some of the more obvious points of convergence between fine medical work and accomplished musicianship. High-level performance in each domain requires motivation, technical mastery, disciplined scholarship, endless practice, personal honesty, professionalism, and the subordination of individual ambitions to the larger purposes of giving care or putting forth an effective performance.

But the most important gratification that derives from my life as both a physician and musician comes from the privileged access to profound aspects of the human experience that each profession provides. What makes me a more complete person and a better physician for being a tuba player is that the music keeps me in touch with the emotional underpinnings of life. It enables me to care.

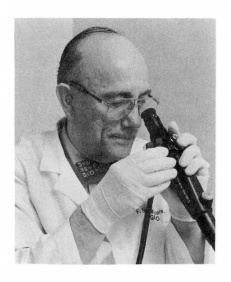

Another gastroenterologist and jazz musician,

NORMAN VICKERS, plays the ukulele, rhythm

guitar, piano, and flute, but his preferred instrument is

the chromatic harmonica, which he has been known to

play for patients in his waiting room. Of the many

similarities between music and medicine, the most

important, Dr. Vickers believes, is the discipline

required of both. He writes that medicine involves

science and art, whereas music is about technique and

feeling "from the heart." In the late 1950s, an intro-

duction to fiber-optic instruments during his training

in gastroenterology led to yet another interest—

photography. These three fields have often merged in

his life and work, creating a unique synthesis.

Jazzdoc

F. Norman Vickers, M.D.

I t has been said that there are more musical physicians than one would expect statistically. To me, this makes sense: both music and medicine are strict disciplines. If someone can learn the twelve major scales, then he or she can probably memorize the twelve cranial nerves or the bones of the foot. Much of medicine, when most effectively practiced, is itself an art. As with music, it exceeds the strictly technical and should be performed from the heart.

Despite my love of making music, I have never had illusions about becoming a professional musician: rather, the idea of becoming a physician stuck with me from about the age of six. On childhood visits to my maternal grandfather, Dr. Cicero Gibson, of Thomson, Georgia, and to my uncle and namesake, Dr. Frank Norman Gibson, I was impressed by their kindliness and warmth and by the respect they received from the community. My childlike logic determined that physicians were somehow special, and I wanted to be like them.

My paternal great-grandfather, Dr. John C. Goodman, was a surgeon in Lee's Army of Virginia. He left Virginia for Georgia in search of a healthier climate for his wife, who apparently suffered from chronic bronchitis. Dr. Goodman set up his new practice in Tifton, Georgia, sharing his stories of the Confederate Army with my father. My great-grandfather was made manifest to me as a child, because my father was among the relatives who inherited instruments from his Confederate medical kit. There were rongeurs for removing bits of bone from the skull, a scalpel, and smaller items. In the mid-1950s, the kit was donated to the Emory University Medical Collection, at which point all the instruments were reunited. Unfortunately, the manual that had been issued with the kit was lost.

I entered Southern Methodist University (SMU) in Dallas in 1949, when scores of World War II veterans were catching up on higher education. Consequently, competition was keen for medical school slots. I had chosen my medical school before my undergraduate school: my grandfather Gibson had graduated from Atlanta Medical College before it merged with several other schools to become the Emory University School of Medicine. Uncle Frank was also an Emory graduate. Hence Emory sounded right for me. But I wanted to go elsewhere for my baccalaureate to avoid spending eight years in the same city. I learned that SMU had a good reputation with Emory, as well as some good football teams: Doak Walker had won the Heisman trophy in 1948 during his junior year there, and that was enough to sell me.

The premed course left little time for electives and outside activities. I did, however, serve as head cheerleader on an all-male squad (this was the 1940s, when a mixed cheerleading team was still a controversial proposition). In my sophomore year, I took physics and organic chemistry, the two toughest courses of my life, far harder than anything I was to study in medical school. These two classes separated the future physicians from the wanna-bes.

Although my schedule afforded no time for music courses, music nonetheless crept into my busy life. During high school, I had taught myself the ukelele, an instrument that gained popularity through Arthur Godfrey's radio and television programs. At SMU, many of the guys had brought their guitars with them. Upon discovering that the top four strings of the six-string guitar were tuned like those of the uke, I became an instant rhythm guitarist!

One dorm mate, a trombonist in the school band, mentioned that Stan Kenton would be playing a concert on campus and that I shouldn't miss it. I had never heard of Stan Kenton, so my friend played me some seventy-eight records of this loud, dissonant big-band music. Kenton, at that time, was controversial among big-band fans, for good reason: his sound was nothing like the easier listening of Benny Goodman or Glenn Miller. Hearing Kenton's wild style and seeing the energy of his young players whetted my appetite for this so-called progressive jazz.

Another influence on my creative side was a family friend named Lester C. Todd, an allergist from Charlotte, North Carolina. On an official trip to the Philippines for the U.S. government, Todd had served as archivist, recording and photographing the flora and fauna. The framed photographs by him that hung in our house piqued my curiosity about taking pictures.

This interest was to prove useful in medical training. In the early 1960s, fiber-optic instruments for gastroenterology were just becoming available, making it easier to confirm diagnoses and document medical findings. In 1963, Dr. Malcolm Stanley, a gastroenterologist who served as my mentor, and I published the first photographic evidence of aspirin gastritis; this condition had been described in 1937, along with an artist's rendering, but twenty-five years later it was still not widely recognized that aspirin could cause significant bleeding in the stomach. The medical film work I have displayed at conventions has included movies as well as still photos taken through the gastroscope.

By the mid-1970s, after about ten years of medical practice, I felt free to devote more time to jazz—and so I joined a band. The Musicians of the Past (also known as the MOPs) played music from the 1920s on and had been doing charity performances since 1957. I played rhythm guitar and, substituting for clarinet parts, the chromatic harmonica. My role model was the great jazz harmonicist Toots Thielemans, who had the knack of playing through a microphone so as to compete with the brass and reeds. Because the MOPs had other guitarists, I concentrated on the chromatic harmonica, eventually taking a few choruses on some tunes. The chromatic harmonica, unlike a standard harmonica, covers three or four octaves: it is actually two diatonic harmonicas built side by side—for example, a C harmonica and a C-sharp harmonica—with a slide that when pressed raises the tone a half-step. Thus all twelve notes of the chromatic scale, a necessity when playing jazz, can be reached.

Although I also play piano, flute, and guitar, the harmonica, by virtue of its size, allows me to work out a tune when my calls are put on hold or when I am stopped in traffic. Sometimes my patients request a tune while I am on rounds in the hospital. This can be a very useful icebreaker: a physician may seem unapproachable within his medical aura, but patients seem comfortable talking with a musician.

In 1983 I helped form the Jazz Society of Pensacola, contributing my office and staff to the effort. The result was the first Pensacola JazzFest, featuring the guitarist Chuck Wayne as a guest among the local jazz talent. The next year Toots Thielemans performed, along with Wayne and the jazz guitarist Laurindo Almeida. Spending time with Thielemans was particularly inspiring for me.

My interests in jazz and photography came together during that first JazzFest. We needed photos for our archives and newsletter, and I was happy to oblige. A few years later I started attending Dick Gibson's Jazz Party in Denver, the "Superbowl" of jazz get-togethers, which was held annually from 1963 to 1992. Every Labor Day weekend, about sixty musicians would present some thirty hours of all-star jazz to more than six hundred patrons, affording many wonderful photographic opportunities. I was eventually invited to contribute photos for use on album covers, and to date my work has appeared on four releases.

For some years I have also been editor of *Federation Jazz,* the newsletter of the American Federation of Jazz Societies. In this capacity, I plan the photographic content of each issue. As advances in technology diminish the challenge of gastrointestinal photography, jazz subjects increasingly fulfill my impulse to photograph. My life would have been the poorer had any one of my means of expression (medical, photographic, or musical) crowded out the others, but I consider myself fortunate in that all three, coming from the heart, have proven complementary, if not synergistic.

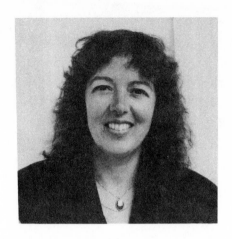

ELAINE BEARER, a gifted musician, gives a lively
account of the fascinating, and sometimes difficult,
path that led her to the practice of medicine. Early in
her career as a composer, pianist, and singer, she
encountered a detour that was to greatly enrich her
life. Dr. Bearer's current work as a research
pathologist and teacher at Brown University has
presented additional challenges. In addition to her
academic duties, once a year she volunteers four weeks
of her time to practice medicine in Guatemala. Her
experiences are a lesson in perseverance and confidence
in the self, and her personal narrative is a testimony to
a life well lived.

Self-Confidence under Siege

Elaine L. Bearer, M.D.

I am currently a professor at Brown University, where I run a biomedical research lab funded by more than a million dollars in federal and private grants. Brown medical students have to pass the course I teach in systemic pathology in order to graduate. I am also involved in medical practice both at home and abroad: during the academic year I participate in the Brown Pathology Residency Program, and for part of each summer I work as a primary-care provider in the Guatemalan highlands. But I also write music, which was all I had set out to do initially. In my compositions, I strive for a sense of classical form while incorporating twentieth-century innovations; they reflect, I hope, the inner voice of my imagination, dreams, and sense of humor.

My accomplishments, however, are not the result of an unbroken string of luck and success. Far from it. The biggest setbacks of my life, and the creative ways in which I dealt with them, proved in the long run to be blessings in disguise.

In 1975 I was in my mid-twenties and well on my way toward accomplishing what I thought were my life's goals. Lone Mountain College, a small liberal arts school in San Francisco, had put me on the faculty of its music department. My position required me to compose music, and because composing felt as essential to me as eating or sleeping, the situation was ideal.

But life had other work for me to do. To escape financial difficulties, Lone Mountain merged with San Francisco University, and my job was eliminated, tenure notwithstanding. This exercise in downsizing, which forced many people in mid-career to start over from scratch, parallels current changes in health-care reimbursements, which affect physicians all over the United States, challenging their income, their style of medical practice, and their job security.

For the next year I couldn't decide what to do. Family obligations prevented me from seeking academic positions outside the Bay area. What's more, I loved San Francisco and felt it was home. I did land another assistant professorship, as a substitute for a professor on a year's sabbatical, but that was only a stopgap measure.

I could have felt trapped: no job, no openings at hand, and no desire or, at the time, freedom to move. At seventeen I had set out on the path that had brought me to this point; from the relatively more mature perspective of twenty-five, I realized that, come what may, contributing to the world, "making a difference," was important to me. Whether I could achieve this through my music only time would tell. But I did know that my temporary job of teaching music to beginners was no answer. Constant exposure to student music, which was either out of tune or artlessly mechanical, risked damage to my inner ear, that place where my creative process germinates.

For a while, self-blame deterred me from reexamining my goals and abilities. If only I had done things differently! Although my troubles stemmed from events entirely outside my control, my feelings had to be acknowledged, expressed, and put to rest before I could summon the courage to move on.

To reestablish my bearings, and my belief in myself, I began by discussing my options with close friends, and beyond that I reconnected with my dearest mentor, who had deeply influenced my life and for whom I had infinite respect and trust. Using most of my savings, I flew to France to visit Nadia Boulanger, who had been my teacher in 1967–68. She was now ninety and in frail health but was spending the summer as usual at the Palace at Fontainebleau. For a week I waited at an eighteenth-century mansion nearby until she was well enough to see me.

Mounting the wide palatial stairs to Boulanger's second-floor apartment, all the love and respect I had felt for her welled up in me again. I had a profound trust that she could rejuvenate my self-confidence, even if she advised me to make some drastic change. Her apartment was filled with vases of fresh flowers and photos in memory of departed family members. Light from the huge seventeenth-century windows glinted off antique silver mirrors. Nadia was sitting near the grand piano in a wheelchair, blind, head drooping to one side, but mentally alert. Her voice was deep and strong when she greeted me. After telling her, in English, about my life in San Francisco and my dilemma, I played one of my pieces on her grand piano. She wore an attentive look and must have constructed the whole score in her mind, for afterward she went over the composition measure by measure, questioning specific notes. What a joy, to be understood so profoundly!

On hearing my second piece, she was moved to tears. At the end, I went over and gently hugged her. I can still feel the gentle pressure of her hands, the weight of the heavy ring with which she used to beat out the rhythm for recalcitrant students. She said, "You don't need me anymore."

But I had come because I did need her! Then I realized what extraordinary praise this was. How could anyone reach a point of not needing her anymore? Even Leonard Bernstein in his fifties had returned for lessons with her. "You have a great gift. You must continue," she told me.

I saw her on several more occasions before my return flight to California. Later, in San Francisco, I received a beautiful letter from Boulanger, reiterating her faith in me and her love of my music. That letter, framed, now hangs in the entry hall of my home in Providence.

Upon my return home, my self-confidence was much improved. Still, there remained the need to restore my sense of personal strength. The best way for me to do this has always been through sports, not in competition but in pursuit of my personal best. I especially like jogging, skiing, and horseback riding, and, lucky for me, that summer my best friend owned a horse. In exchange for mucking out the stall, I got to ride. Mounds and mounds of smelly hay and many sore muscles later, my sense of personal strength returned.

I chose to become a physician and entered medical school at the University of California at San Francisco in 1977. My biomedical studies were directed toward scientific research and medicine. During my residency, I trained in pathology. Currently we are experimenting in my laboratory with novel methods of putting single genes into the chromosomes of bone marrow stem cells, with the hope of developing gene therapy.

I feel that medicine helps only the relatively few patients one can see, whereas research holds the potential to benefit countless people. Still, fulfilling a duty to society cannot substitute for the pleasure that comes with healing a person. Hence I have been extraordinarily fortunate in being able to donate my medical skills, rusty as they are, every summer in the Guatemalan highlands. Originally a few physician friends and I made this trip to volunteer our services, at our own expense. Since then, our annual journey has turned into the Brown University Elective Clerkship, a program that allows medical students from all over the country to earn medical school credits through Brown and at the same time contribute their services where they are sorely needed.

Yet through all else I have never stopped writing music. And at this point, who can say whether music or medicine will prove my more important contribution. Some friends maintain that composing is my most valuable occupation; others, that without the distraction of music, my work in science would be to much greater effect. I am afraid that this will have to remain a moot point, because abandoning music would be unthinkable.

Over the years, my life has been tested in many ways, but I have gradually learned to appreciate challenges. Mistakes, for example, certainly feel adversarial and can make one feel uncomfortable, but they can also be unique openings for new ideas. Sometimes, when playing a musical work in progress, I will accidentally hit a different note from what was written. But this "mistake" may in fact sound better and may give me ideas about incorporating further "wrong" notes. This kind of mistake has opened my mind to possibilities that otherwise would never have occurred to me.

Much the same can happen in the lab. An experiment, though performed well, may not produce the expected result. Although this may be discouraging at first, the experiments that do not work can produce the most significant discoveries, as long as the researcher is patient and observant enough to see what has really been revealed. This has been documented over and over again in the history of science.

Another setback in my career worked to the general scientific good when my initial proposal for funding from the National Institutes of Health was turned down. But in switching to other projects, I discovered something seminal, namely, that in addition to microtubules, actin can also act as tracks for organelle transport in axons. This discovery, which would never have come about had my first proposal been approved, has led to new insights about Alzheimer's disease. One can never predict how persistence will pay off.

In 1996, this was demonstrated to me yet again in a musical context. I had written a composition as a sixty-fifth birthday gift for John Nicholls, a great friend and mentor since my medical student days and a distinguished neurophysiologist whose groundbreaking studies of axonal regeneration have inspired generations. I sent a digitally processed tape of my composition to Composer's Recordings, Inc. (CRI), a producer of compact disks, but according to their rejection letter, my submission was not up to their standards. Friends assured me that my work did indeed have merit, so I decided to turn my disappointment into an opportunity. I went to New York and insisted on meeting the director at CRI to discuss why he had refused my tape and how I could either improve it or market it elsewhere. Taking him to lunch cost me nearly a week's pay, but once he understood that I was open to his opinion of my music, he relaxed and gave me a good deal of indispensable advice. My next submission met with immediate acceptance, and the resulting CD is now available. At a popular record store, I've even found a divider in the classical bins with my name on it, right between Bartók and Beethoven.

Mistakes and adversity, I've discovered, can open more doors than first-time success—if they are handled with insight and inspiration. Learning from error without losing self-esteem, rethinking long-term goals when appropriate, talking with mentors, friends, family, and knowledgeable specialists, and being persistent have all helped me grow and get to know myself better. Indeed, these have been my guidelines for getting the most out of life.

Part 3

Literature

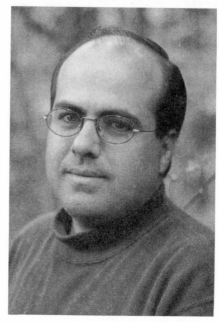

Jorge Arroyo

Poetry and healing are "powerfully united in the human consciousness," asserts RAFAEL CAMPO, as he recounts how poetry has permeated the art of healing from antiquity to the present, serving as "its vital partner, its sister art." Poetry existed before medicine and needs no justification to medical practitioners once they understand that poetic expression pictures the deep resources of the human heart and spirit. A gifted writer of fiction, essays, and poetry, Campo finds his avocation an antidote to the hate and fear that arose from his early painful childhood experiences as an outsider, a gay Cuban adolescent in an unsympathetic America.

A Prescription for Poetry

Rafael Campo, M.D.

The poet is humankind's first healer, so it has long been perplexing to me that my own engagement with verse should define me as an outsider in relation to today's medical world. It is usually not my patients who are suspicious of poetry; they are in fact the very ones who are searching desperately for the right words to help them make sense of their afflictions. Rather, some of my physician-colleagues distrust the poetic, especially those who might think they have all the relevant information fully explained in their sterile odds ratios and neatly tabulated significant p values. I sometimes wonder whether they cite only lists of references from glossy medical journals when their patients ask them what they should read to learn more about their illnesses. Perhaps they reject the poem as being too primitive or confessional, not at all "sexy" and far too subjective, perpetually unfunded by the National Institutes of Health, certainly not a basis for academic promotion, and ultimately quite unquantifiable. I wonder, because I myself once believed in the supremacy of scientific discourse as a definitive answer to human suffering and resisted what, at the time, I would have called poetry's pathetic attempts to coax me away from vastly more glamorous, productive, and rigorous pursuits.

Yet through the ages, poetry and healing have remained powerfully united in the human consciousness. The richness of historical examples that bespeak the profound connection between poetic expression and the therapeutic alliance of healer and patient is astonishing. Perhaps most ancient are the numerous Native American traditions in which breath and incantation were employed by medicine men or shamans to cast out illness; many accounts exist of dramatic cures effected by these practices, some of which survive on far-flung reservations to this day. The importance of the relationship between expressive language and healing was explicitly represented in the theology of the ancient Greeks: Apollo was the revered god of both poetry and sunlight, his symbols both the gentle lyre and the proud staff, his children the graceful Muses, who inspired poets, and the noble Aesculapius, the great healer. In the more recent Judeo-Christian tradition, Jesus is shown healing with words, words that in their wisdom and concision sing like purest poetry. Even in our own age, at the beginning of modern American medicine, the fundamental link between literary work and medical practice may be glimpsed: Dr. Benjamin Rush, whose Pennsylvania Hospital of 1810 eventually became the main model for today's sprawling, centralized medical centers, included in his original design a grand library where patients could read books prescribed to them by their doctors.

Why, then, has the current medical culture so roundly ignored what for millennia has been considered, in diverse civilizations and traditions, its vital partner, its sister art? This question becomes all the more urgent and intriguing as the medical profession confronts the explosive technological expansion fueled by its unquenchable passion for basic science research but also the financial imperatives of managed care that pressure clinicians to see more patients in less time, while injudiciously employing all that glittering new technology. When I give lectures and readings at medical centers around the country, one of the most common questions I am asked by other doctors is an impatient one: How can one advocate teaching and thinking about literary matters in the face of the terrible upheavals that are ruining our profession, when so much else, from pharmacologic advances and novel genetic techniques to health-economics seminars and time-management strategies, needs to be taught and engaged by our profession? In response, I echo what I hear in other venues, in bookstores, English departments, and humanities centers, where laypeople poignantly share stories of how little their physicians *hear* them these days and express their belief that physicians need poetry just as they do, both to help them become better listeners and to nourish their spirits.

So there is a utilitarian value in placing poetry alongside medicine. I find sometimes that my defense of poetry to physician-colleagues—and even to the outside world, which in many quarters remains surprisingly indifferent to poetry—often relies on the most practical of arguments: that poetry is necessary because it can help model empathic relationships between care providers and patients, that it can teach an alternate anatomy of the heart totally neglected in the standard course on gross anatomy, that it should be read before medical rounds to remind us of our patients' and our own humanity. Such a pragmatic view paradoxically can diminish the value of poetry for its own sake, which has so long flourished outside medicine and the other professions, creating distinct communities and traditions of its own. Poetry need not be justified, and my intent here is not to rationalize it. I recognize and resist the scientist's impulse in me to analyze the poem into oblivion or to predicate its worth on a system of beliefs that poetry itself predates.

Although I could never calculate to the third decimal place any specific dimensions or parameters pertaining to a poem, nor would I want to, I *can* speak to some of the principles that give rise to its therapeutic force. Indeed, to begin with, its refusal to be so analyzed is central to its mysterious power: to read or to hear a poem is to enter entirely into the voice of another, to relinquish control and to allow oneself to be guided from without. Parodoxically, poetry is at once utterly subjective and yet ultimately universalizing. It catalyzes the exchange between one body and another almost exactly like it, reconstituting one set of experiences with the lifeblood of the participant heart. The rhythm of the breathing lungs or the beating heart, those elusive targets of our stethoscopes, ultrasound probes, X rays, and ever more costly and sophisticated diagnostic technologies, can be startlingly bared in an eloquent poem. As such, poetry truly is the ideal medium for exploring empathy, that most inexplicable and unquantifiable of all our human capacities. Poetry is there when the last of our gizmos and gadgets fails us; it gave meaning to life long before we ever had such fancy toys; it helps us gauge that which cannot be assayed in the blood, to see what cannot be imagined.

The Couple

Releasing his determined grip, he lets
her take the spoon; the cube of cherry Jell-O
teeters on it, about to drop as if
no precipice were any steeper, no

oblivion more final. Earlier
today, he hemorrhaged, the blood so fast
a torrent that it splattered onto her.
She washed herself, unwillingly it seemed,

perhaps not wanting to remove what was
his ending life from where it stained her skin.
I watch them now, the way they love across
the gap between them that their bodies make:

how cruel our life-long separation seems.
The ward keeps narrowing itself to that
bright point outside his door—the muffled screams
along a hallway to the absolute—

and as I turn away from them it's not
their privacy, or even my beginning shame
I wish I could escape. It is the light,
the awful light of what we know must come.

Rafael Campo

The primacy of poetry as a modality for healing is further illustrated, albeit more anecdotally, by some of my own experiences in becoming a doctor. The process was an arduous one for me. As a child, I first sensed acutely the fracture of my differences from those around me—I felt that my dark ethnicity and my sexuality set me apart. My impulse to repair those divisions initially took the form of an irresistible desire to write poetry. The act of putting pen to paper, much more imaginable than piercing a person's vein with a needle, opened up a vast internal geography to me, a body whose limitations were imposed not by physiology (as I would later learn in medical school) but by ignorance and silence. Of course, I knew the body was hard-wired for pain, and that a punch in the jaw could send blinding electrical shocks to the brain. Yet I discovered quickly that those same pathways could conduct images and sounds that might modulate or reconfigure pain, producing instead a kind of beauty that was an antidote to hate and fear. Poetic language was therefore my first salve, what I applied to the wound of my potentially disfiguring identities. Not until much later did the notion of my becoming a doctor evolve, and then it was mostly an outgrowth of, or a wish to refine, what I had learned was possible through the poem.

As time passed, formal poetry appealed to me ever more intensely, because in mastering its rules and structures I felt a kind of control over the process of living in my world of disparate human identities. I could stanch the flow of blood from my own injured mouth with the stitchlike quality of rhymes; I could gallop away from danger or dance with joy in my crude syllabics. Rather than invading me forcibly, poetry pushed into me gently, viscerally, sexually, the way I wanted to be touched and entered. The rhythms of love-making seized me in the sonnets I read, instantly curing me of my self-loathing, teaching me, as I thrilled to their gorgeousness, that in truth my erotic nature was no different from anyone else's and that the body's most pleasurable expressions could be communicated in a catholic code of meaning. As for the question of my ethnicity, I could also rejoice in recognizing the music of my Spanish heritage infusing the villanelles and sestinas I relished. The kinetics of my Cuban father's conversations with his family were not something to be ashamed of after all; on the contrary, they could be harnessed in the fireworks of great poetry.

What was most curative about poetry was how unabashedly democratic it was; no matter what, I lived in America, the free country that had saved my parents from oppression. When I felt unwelcome in a classroom or on a playground, I could find sustenance and sanctuary in the timeless words of Walt Whitman and William Carlos Williams, who each tended to the deep scars of their times with bandages and poetry and who created a living body of words that reached me in my middle-class immigrant suburban bedroom. Their life-sustaining ministrations made possible the vigorous and vibrant society that later produced the likes of Allen Ginsberg and Adrianne Rich, and Elizabeth Bishop and Robert Frost, poets I read with almost equal reverence, poets who taught me how I could exist in my own "body electric" despite the hatred (of foreigners, of homosexuals) to which I was so often exposed. Instead of the psychiatrist who might propose to "cure" me of my differentness, in place of the pediatrician whose vaccination against polio might give me the disease itself, I discovered a healing well of voices in which I heard plainly echoed my own humanity. My mind's words, my body's rhythms, my tongue's movement, my heart's song: poetry was all of these, my naturally occurring remedy for all kinds of sorrow, drawn from the mythical fountain of youth that my Spanish ancestors had sought in the perilous New World so many centuries ago.

Despite my early affinity to the poem as the expressive soul of a nation struggling to be born out of so many rhythms and races and languages, a struggle I myself was embodying on a much smaller scale, hard medicine soon barged into my consciousness as an alternative mode of understanding humanity. In high school and college, as I became more and more socialized in the obligate culture of rage and violence of young American males—a disturbing world that ranks contact sports above conversation, keg parties over Kirkegaard, and hard rock ahead of Prufrock—I began to imagine that medical school might be the means by which I could subdue all the conflict within me, rather than making peace with myself through poetry. I fantasized that the white coat I would receive in medical school might sanitize my swarthy skin, that the staccato of medical jargon barked from my mouth might be the most irrefutable testimony that I had mastered English, that the brutality of the medical training I would endure might toughen me up and finally straighten out my queerness. I also saw that I could make a killing in medicine, my large paycheck a measure of my masculinity, my expensive car and my well-appointed home the most compelling and satisfying expressions of my American dreams. Poetry soon faded quietly and rather quaintly into the background of my intellectual life.

One cannot really know human suffering until one has stared into its eyes: all the poetry I had read seemed terribly distant, and even irrelevant, once I embarked on my medical training. By the end of my third year at Harvard Medical School, I had witnessed what I believed was every kind of atrocity imaginable. My first patient during my internal medicine rotation was an elderly retarded man whose family had forgotten to give him water for two weeks; I wanted to be as fascinated by his lethal serum sodium level of 198 as my supervising intern and resident were, but what struck me most was how he bleated "Mary had a little lamb" over and over to himself whenever I came to draw his blood. I wanted to get excited about the complicated facial fracture I saw on the X rays of a battered woman but found that I kept hearing instead the soft noise her husband made as he tapped his foot impatiently outside the examining room. The child of a drug-using mother arrived in the emergency room one night, having ingested some cocaine the mother must have left on the kitchen table; as I grappled with the complex pathophysiology of the boy's seizures, I grew mesmerized by his mother's singing to him through the long night. In any of these and countless other incidents, as much as the science pertaining to each case intrigued me, I could not so easily fractionate the protein from the sweating, aching muscles of the whole organism; I could not so capably isolate the genetic defect that caused the pain of my patients' cancers; I could not separate the arrhythmia apparent on an electrocardiogram, its risings and fallings like an orchestral score waiting to be animated, from the actual music the integrated body made.

As I learned dutifully about the medical problems of my patients, I also strained against the built-in limitations of scientific knowledge. I saw that I could not avoid confronting the many levels of meaning sounded by human suffering by stultifying my imagination with cold facts; I had shown a kind of hubris in pretending that I could read my patients as dispassionately as I did the dense textbooks containing precious information about their illnesses. I knew that most of my patients were helped by certain medical interventions, yet I saw some who were not and some who were even harmed. All of them needed me to understand their afflictions not only in terms of cells and viscera and organ systems but also in the language of the spirit that inhabited what seemed such fragile and temporary physical structures. Gradually, I rediscovered the transcendent power of poetry, which could move and speak after rigor mortis had set in, which could console in the face of anger and denial, which could rekindle communication in the apoplectic, which could make sex safe again, which could contain all that the heart could—not in the limited physical dimensions of its chamber but in its limitlessness as the seat of our souls.

Yesterday I saw a patient named Alan, a young man about my age who is ten years from his diagnosis of testicular cancer. He'd come in because he was concerned about having coughed up some blood, just a little, which I was trying to interpret as merely bronchitis, trying to explain away as nothing serious. As we talked about his symptoms and what they might mean, reviewing his yearly alpha fetoprotein (AFP) and human chorionic gonadotropin (HCG) levels and studying his hila on the ghostly chest X ray, he suddenly interrupted me apologetically and asked if he could change the subject. He complimented me on my most recent book of poetry, which he had read, and wondered whether someday I would write something about him. My frustration and embarrassment must have been apparent, because before I knew it I was back to expounding on my medical diagnosis, intent on reassuring him. I sent him on his way with a prescription for antibiotics, instructions to call if his symptoms worsened, and a promise to call him in a few days with the results of the blood tests I had ordered.

It wasn't until later that day, when I was at home surrounded by my books and journals, that I suddenly realized how terrified Alan must have been, how he must have been thinking he would be dead soon. In my fluorescently lit office, I had assessed him as disease-free for ten years, with flat AFP levels, and so for all intents and purposes "cured"—and besides, I had three other patients waiting to be seen. As I admired the sun painting the clouds red outside my window, a line of Marilyn Hacker's came to me, from a sequence of sonnets, love poems, that she wrote about life after her treatment for breast cancer—"The setting sun looks terribly like blood." I realized in that startling image, and the flood of associations it engendered, what Alan might be seeing in every sunset: that he would always be living with testicular cancer, that all the sophisticated tumor markers in the world could not liberate him, that his own blood would always deeply unnerve him. I took out a clean sheet of paper and started to write. The poem that took shape has not cured him of testicular cancer, in the way the surgeon's knife may have; the words on the page will not change the result of the blood tests I ordered, and they are not another prescription for the chemotherapeutic agents that I hope will never be indicated again. The poem is simply the small thing that Alan wanted.

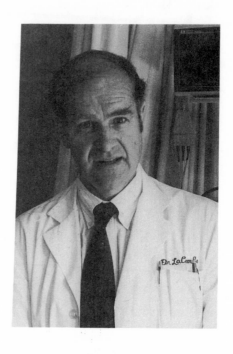

MICHAEL A. LACOMBE has practiced internal medicine in Maine for more than twenty years. But he has been a writer much longer. Frustrated by the rejection of his essays by leading medical journals, he began to write fiction, becoming the first writer to publish fictional pieces about doctors and patients in scientific publications. When he left his practice some years ago to write full-time, he discovered how closely linked his patients were to his Muse. He now combines his writing career with part-time practice. Dr. LaCombe still makes housecalls.

Getting Famous

Michael A. LaCombe, M.D.

Some years ago now, having become increasingly frustrated with the decline of traditional medicine and having always turned to writing to vent such frustrations, I began to write what I considered to be learned essays. These essays examined the evils of malpractice, the idiocy of Medicare, the meddling of business into medicine, and the loss of humanism in our profession—topics I felt worthy of publication. I sent them to various leading medical journals and, ready to change the world with my writing, waited for the phone to ring, waited for the interviews, the television appearances.

The letters of rejection came as a faucet dripping in the night, annoying, incessant, sleep-depriving. I revised each rejected piece, gave it to a friend or partner to read, and revised some more, resubmitting each to a different journal, each with an increasingly strident and supplicating cover letter. Still, the essays were rejected, so quickly in some cases that I began to doubt they had even been read. I was angry, of course, as are all rejected writers, and with the rest of them thought all editors fools, all journals worthless. Then I tried the popular intellectual magazines— *Harper's, Atlantic Monthly,* the *New Yorker*—and in most instances never received a reply at all. What was going on? I wondered. Was this a conspiracy against Truth? Didn't they know I was a doctor, a graduate of Harvard even?

I began to look at my predicament as any internist would: as a problem to be solved. I proceeded to examine every essay and editorial in every journal I could lay my hands on. In every instance, I found the author to be an academician with title, academic rank, and university address after his or her name. And here I was, a general internist, a country doctor *practicing* medicine no less, in a remote town in rural Maine, expecting to be published along with these icons of medicine.

Well, I thought, here's what I would do: I decided to write the pieces as fiction, always with a message, but deans and department chairs and assorted glitterati of my own invention would do my talking for me. I had only two rules: I would never disparage the practicing physician, and I would neither exploit Medicine nor cause the reader to fear my profession. My first piece, an allegory about Medicare's senseless rules, written in the form of government takeover of French bakeries, was accepted by a major medical journal almost immediately. I felt entitled for weeks, anticipated recognition on the streets of larger cities, that sort of thing. I wrote more stories and sent them in — in fact, I couldn't seem to write them fast enough. Every day, a patient, a colleague, or a clinical dilemma sparked an idea. And every story was accepted. Miraculously, in Claude Bennett at the *American Journal of Medicine* and in the Fletchers at the *Annals of Internal Medicine,* I had found kindred spirits.

There were rejections, of course. From the former editor of one preeminent journal: "I am sorry we cannot accept your piece. It is too literary." And from its present editor: "Your piece seems to be fiction. I am sorry we have no one on our editorial staff qualified to review it." Upon sending a manuscript about the ethical dilemma of duty to patient versus duty to law, I received this reply: "I am sorry we are forced to reject your piece. Half of our editorial board said they would publish it only if it is fiction; the other half, only if it is non-fiction. Which is it?"

But the reception by physician-readers of fiction in medical journals more than compensated for these few rejections. Letters arrived from around the world. Practitioners wrote to me about reaffirmation; a doctor in Siberia told me things were not all that different there; a medical student in Manila wrote that the stories persuaded him to return to his original inclination to study medicine. A radiologist in Prague invited me over for a beer—and we have since become close friends.

With this colossal good luck—predictable publication and tangible acceptance—I caught fire. I wrote every morning without fail from five until seven and then went off to my job at the hospital. Writing in this way gave my whole life a new dimension. I saw patients differently. I became more sensitive to them, understood them more deeply, partly because I was looking for the story and partly because writing does that to you. I wrote only because it was fun, exciting, because it energized me, made me a better doctor, gave me a tingle at the nape of my neck, led me to self-discovery, taught me how I felt about things. It all seemed so easy. I was yet to learn that writing, serious writing, is far more difficult than medicine.

The first few stories were easy; they almost wrote themselves. A pulmonologist, playing with a computer, taps into artificial intelligence and loses a debate over nuclear armament. A fat, balding history professor argues successfully against three sleek and learned scientists over the sacred nature of patient confidentiality, with three humanoid robots as judges. A Jewish scientist and professor of pediatrics covers for the hospital staff at Christmas and tells a dying girl a story of Christ.

Then, the writing became more difficult. At one level, I was competing with myself and my past successes. At another level, I wanted to be better, found I couldn't draw characters well, couldn't layer my messages, couldn't hook and trick my readership very well—those busy, distracted physicians with their stacks of journals. My dialogue was artificial or dishonest, as we writers would say, and my narrative, flat and lifeless. Neither seminars nor books on writing resolved these weaknesses.

At this juncture, a semiretired English professor came into my life. I had been asked by our surgeon to do a preoperative consultation on this man, who was to have major and potentially debilitating surgery the next morning. I told him, after some analysis, that he didn't necessarily need it, that there was a nonsurgical way out of this and that I would be happy to help him along. He would take me up on it, he said, and work with me, but he had poor insurance coverage and would have to barter with me for his office visits. He knew that I was a part-time writer, having read some of my pieces in a regional magazine. He would, in exchange for my medical care, help me with my writing. I could use it, he explained. His brutal honesty was to become the benchmark of our relationship. I could rely upon his telling me exactly what was so. It was the best deal I ever made.

Our arrangement was this: I'd mail him a manuscript, call him a week later, and set a date to see him. Always we met at his home, tucked in the woods adjacent to the private school where he had taught for forty-five years, where he still believed that a C was a perfectly adequate, average grade.

"Show, don't tell," he would say, and "Choose one, don't give me a list." And "Adjectives diminish. Always. Adverbs weaken verbs." And this: "Read that sentence . . . no, read it aloud. There now. Doesn't that sound silly?" And this, his grandest compliment to me ever: "That's a pretty good sentence. Nearly perfect, I'd say." (After ten years and a hundred more stories, I can still remember the sentence to which he was referring.)

He taught me anticlimax with Edna St. Vincent Millay's sonnets, dialogue through Hemingway's stories, characterization by Victor Hugo's wonderful example, voice from Frank O'Connor. Voice— most important of all.

It was all still fun.

It was at this point, too, that I discovered the Muses; I learned that they exist, that they are shy and reclusive (as a writer must be) and will run from you when you most urgently seek them. And I found that when the Muses do whisper to you, they often do so in the most oblique, tangential of ways.

I became, if not spotted at Forty-second and Broadway, well then, somewhat recognized within my profession. There were invitations to give readings, present grand rounds, do visiting professorships. And largely through this recognition as a storyteller came that most heady invitation of all: to become a director of the American Board of Internal Medicine. That four-year tenure was to be followed by election as a regent in internal medicine's national organization, the American College of Physicians. It was beyond my grandest dreams. Merely because of telling stories, I had achieved a position of power, an opportunity to change, if not the world, then medicine's decline. I thought I had become somebody.

But for the writer part of me, it was nearly death. I was no longer writing. I was too busy being famous. More than that, these organizations, with their adversarial form of debate, their crushing of ideas, the hierarchical form of decision making by decree, the dearth of thought and lack of joy in mere thinking, the reluctance to share possible solutions, were devastating for the writer in me.

Writers, after all, think and write by free association much of the time, with assistance from Jung's collective unconscious. Instead, at the board level, I was getting a hard lesson in what Zeuxis taught twenty-four hundred years ago: "Criticism comes easier than craftsmanship."

To compound the malady, I had left the practice of medicine ostensibly to write full-time but found that I could not. In leaving medicine, I had left that front-row seat in the drama of life, left that spark that fires the creative energy in the physician-writer. I had forsaken experience for fame. Now I could understand why writers traveled endlessly, fought in civil wars, and lived in garret flats in Paris. For experience. Medicine, I learned, gave me more than experience, more than simply a cast of characters; it offered up a welter of stories of the human experience and plotlines one could never dream up. Medicine put me in touch with humanity and its suffering and granted me glimpses of the courage, dignity, and integrity of another. What I had encountered every day, other writers desperately coveted, continually searched for, and often never found.

And so I went back to medicine, back to full-time practice, returned to the familiar conflicts of the physician-writer: when to find time, how to set priorities, whether the written page can ever be more important than the sick patient, how far might I stretch the patience of my wife and children? I discovered the Solzhenitsyn Phenomenon, so integral to the life of the physician-writer: Solzhenitsyn never wrote a word until he was thrown in prison.

But I also went back with a deeper appreciation of medicine and a deeper understanding of how and what it means to take care of patients. I found that the doctor needs to give patients stories as well as take them, needs to be a character rather than merely hunt for them.

I became convinced that patients want emotion from their doctor, and empathy, and do not want providers, do not want to be simply clients.

When I left medicine, it was partly, I thought, to pursue the higher art of writing. I believed then that writing was far more difficult than medicine. I no longer believe so. Certainly physician-writers face that familiar personal dichotomy of all writers: one's creative side always judged harshly, and usually unfairly, by one's critical, analytical side. But good doctors face that too, every day. Good doctors take their work home rather than punch out, talk to their spouses about that long art, that difficult decision, that all-too-brief life. Good doctors sleep with that dichotomy. Yes, writers are faced more than ever with a public for whom magazines write on a sixth-grade reading level, and with editors who desire sex and sensation more than they do art and grace, and with agents whose only focus is money. But isn't that aspect of the writing life simply a metaphor for the doctor's life in the era of managed care?

The writing life is one of continual rejection—it goes with the territory. Accept it, one is advised, or leave. But so is a life in medicine. I mean the life of the generalist, who takes care of each patient to the very limits of his or her ability, who stays current for the sake of the patient rather than for want of an attitude at conferences, and who is nevertheless scrutinized by those who have narrowed their professional lives to such a degree as to be beyond reproach—who say themselves, and through their educated patients: "If you're so good, what are you doing in Bridgton, Maine? Please, before you go any further, call my cardiologist." There is, I think you will agree, the hint of rejection there.

Writing is both art and science. As a science, one must learn the craft. How do you hook the reader? How do keep yourself, the writer, so far in the background so as not to be noticed? How can you catch and paint a character so unforgettably that the reader feels he or she has created that person himself? What does it really mean, to show, not tell? And as an art, one must find one's voice, connect with that collective unconscious, and if you are fortunate enough, occasionally hear the Muses. You must develop in yourself what Hemingway said was essential for every true writer: a built-in bullshit detector. Writing is not, in other words, what you will get to when you finally have the time.

With medicine, the science is difficult enough. It keeps changing. But medicine's art is harder still and will always be essential to the care of patients, whatever else someone may try to tell you. It is this art that is the more difficult side of medicine, more difficult even than writing. You have to love people and *want* to care for them. You have to understand their frailties and faults, as well as your own. You have to give of yourself while you are getting that history and reveal yourself even as you disrobe and touch that other human being. You need to learn when to be paternal (or maternal) and when to give it up, when to be adamant and when to understand, when to be honest and when to lie, how to be right without being arrogant, how to give patients everything they need but not everything they want, and how to know the difference.

The art of medicine, you see, is to connect with patients. And after twenty years of practice, I am only beginning to learn to do so. But writing has certainly helped me get there.

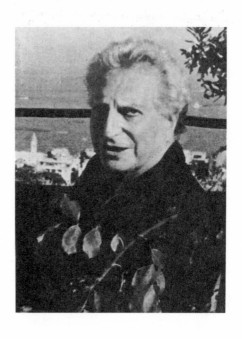

CARLO LEVI (1902–75) left behind not only a
legacy of social justice and political involvement but a
rich collection of paintings and writings. Because he is
so little known in the United States, we asked Dr.
Harvey Mandell, a retired internist, to write about
Levi the physician, painter, senator, humanist, and
antifascist voice. This account will, we hope, encourage
the reader to delve into the remarkable writings of
this equally remarkable artist.

Carlo Levi, M.D.

AN ANTIFASCIST PHYSICIAN

Harvey Mandell, M.D.

Carlo Graziadio Levi, physician, painter, writer, antifascist, prisoner, exile, senator, and humanist, was born in Turin in 1902 to a Jewish family well established in Italy. Although he received a degree from the medical school in that city in 1924, he had already decided before graduation to abandon medicine for painting. After serving as a medical assistant at the university and spending a requisite year in the military as a medical sublieutenant, he believed he was through with medical practice forever.

During his student days Levi had been part of a group of artists influenced by Piero Gobetti, a liberal socialist writer and politician. Levi wrote for Gobetti's journal *Rivoluzione Liberale,* and Gobetti wrote the first review of Levi's painting in *Ordine Nuovo* while Levi was still a medical student. It was a dangerous association: by the age of twenty-five, Gobetti was dead, killed by fascists. During Levi's last year in medical school, his portrait of his father was exhibited in Turin, and the next year, another family portrait, *Arcadia,* was shown at the Venice Biennial.

Like so many artists in the 1920s, Levi headed for

I wish to thank A. Peter Rinaudo, M.D., Estelle Gilson, George Trone, Eric Levregeois, and David Ward for their contributions and their translations.

Paris, where he set up a studio and absorbed the cultural movements of that period. Under the influence of Georges Seurat, whose work Levi admired, his stroke relaxed, his landscapes and figures took on more light and clarity, and his colors became more intense. While in Paris, he helped form "Sei Pittore di Torino" (Six Painters of Turin), a group united in its opposition to the nationalistic academy of the Novocento, the movement responsible for creating the art of fascist Italy. By the end of the decade, Levi's paintings were being widely exhibited, both locally and internationally.

Returning to Italy, Carlo Levi held fast to his antifascist views, and in 1931, with the brothers Carlo and Nello Roselli, he joined the Justice and Liberty movement, most of whose members were nonreligious Jews whose formal faith had been replaced by social awareness and a sense of justice. The movement, which included Russian-born Leone Ginzburg, a fiery leftist and antifascist activist, did not remain unknown to the authorities for long. On the basis of incriminating evidence, Levi and other members were arrested for conspiring against the regime. Levi's paintings of this period include *Portrait of Leone Ginzburg,* who is depicted with red hands (Ginzburg was later tortured by the Germans), and *Self-Portrait with Bloodied Shirt.*

The first half of the 1930s brought arrests and rearrests. A search of the apartment of his friend and fellow writer Cesare Pavesi turned up materials linking Levi and others with leftists. Brought to trial, they were found guilty and sentenced to prison. At the same time that Levi was politically out of favor with Italian authorities, his paintings were being displayed at the Jeu de Paume in Paris and his art was gaining increased acceptance in art circles throughout France.

Incarcerated in Rome at the felicitously named Regina Coeli (Queen of the Sky) prison, Levi was later freed in an amnesty. He failed, however, to keep his pen capped and his mouth closed. For these indiscretions he found himself exiled to Gagliano, a village south of Eboli, near the instep of Italy's boot. The area was so deep in the country and so desolate that, according to the peasants there, no hope existed, for Christ had stopped at Eboli.

Other political prisoners were already there when Levi arrived, but they were not permitted to communicate with one another in any way. Levi wondered aloud to the authorities how two men sharing a plate of spaghetti could be such a danger to the state, but the rule was never lifted.

Some years later, during the war, while hidden in a house in Florence, Levi wrote his magnum opus, *Christo si fermato a Eboli* (*Christ Stopped at Eboli*), which earned him status as a writer equal to his status as a painter. In this work he described the peasants he had encountered:

> "We're not Christians" the *condatini* (peasants) say. "Christ stopped short of here, at Eboli." Christian, in their way of speaking, means "human being," and this almost proverbial phrase that I have so often heard them repeat may be no more than the expression of a hopeless feeling of inferiority. "We're not Christians, we're not human beings; we're not thought of as men but simply as beasts, beasts of burden, or even less than beasts, mere creatures of the wild. They at least live for better or for worse, like angels or demons, in a world of their own, while we have to submit to the world of Christians, beyond the horizon, to carry its weight and to stand comparison to it. . . . Christ never came this far, nor did time, nor the individual soul, nor hope, nor the relation of cause to effect, nor reason nor history."

After the war this extraordinary, beautifully written book was published and quickly translated into a number of languages. Fifty years later, this story is still worth reading, for Levi's description of the human condition of the condatini in that village of despair remains fresh and pertinent.

During his exile in Gagliano, Levi had no wish to use his medical training. But the villagers soon learned that the new arrival was a physician and went to him almost at once to announce that one of the villagers was extremely sick. For the first of many times Levi explained that he had not practiced medicine for years and suggested that there must be another doctor on call in the village. Despite Levi's reservations about his clinical abilities, he was persuaded to attend the patient. The man was moribund from malaria, a local scourge, and died soon thereafter.

It was not long before Levi met one of the two village doctors, the uncle of the fascist mayor. This local physician did not welcome a new doctor in the village, until he realized that Levi did not plan to practice medicine. The village doctor obviously lacked any useful medical knowledge, although he tried hard to resurrect a few scientific terms during the conversation. His universal treatment was quinine. He was kind enough to warn Dr. Levi: "Don't take anything from a woman. Neither wine nor coffee; nothing to eat or drink. They would be sure to put a philter or love potion in it. . . . Don't accept anything from the peasant women. These potions are dangerous. Unpleasant to the taste, in fact disgusting. Do you want to know what they are made of? Blood, ca-ta-menial blood."

Later the other doctor in the village sought him out, mostly to find out if he was to have a new competitor. Even more ignorant than the first, he had a slightly different view of health matters in the village. "The peasants pay no attention to us. They don't even call us when they are sick. Or else they won't pay. They want to be looked after and not to pay for it. But they'll find out. They don't trust the pharmacy. Of course there's not a complete stock of drugs, but we can make one thing do for another. If there's no morphine, then we use apomorphine." The pharmacy, such as it was, was managed by this man's two daughters, neither of whom had had any training relevant to the job. The laboratories and X-ray units of the large urban areas remained inaccessible to the peasants.

Soon, the peasant women were bringing their children to Levi's door for medical advice. Despite his continued protestations of incompetence and his wish not to practice medicine, the women refused to move until he saw their children and counseled them about their health. He slowly realized that they saw in him someone who could not be worse than the village doctors and who treated them like human beings, unlike the local gentry. Although the peasants knew Levi's first patient had died, they did not blame him; rather, they had been warmed by his attempt to comfort the dying man and his family. Although Levi wanted only to paint, it became impossible for him to refuse their pleas for any shred of compassionate care.

The superstitions, ignorance, and belief in witchcraft of the peasants troubled Levi at first, but with his rising respect and affection for them, he learned to work around these obstacles. This situation is not so different from American medicine sixty years later, when so many Americans see their personal physicians, while also engaging in alternative medicine, filling themselves with nostrums, and consulting chiropractors and naturopaths. Had Charles Dickens been Italian, he might have written of these peasants with humor and irony; Levi describes them with straightforward affection and respect, although with no less realism than Dickens.

His medical practice was consuming, but not to the point of precluding his painting. He often set his easel in the shade of an olive tree near the edge of the village, waiting for the rising of the moon, so big it looked almost artificial. That overhead moon reminded him of his months in a windowless prison cell devoid of such beauty. Levi also painted local scenes and sensitive portraits of the villagers.

In 1936, in celebration of the glorious victory over Ethiopia, Levi was freed as part of a general amnesty and immediately moved to Rome. More exhibitions of his paintings followed, and more anti-fascist articles by him appeared in print. He became a principal in the newly opened Galleria, which proved a favorite among young Roman artists, but rising anti-Semitism caused its closing after a few years. Levi left for France, where he continued his political activities and art. Two years later, on returning to Italy, he was again arrested but released. For the rest of the war, he remained hidden in Florence, writing, painting, and participating in the resistance against the Nazi-fascist alliance.

After the war, exhibitions of his paintings, watercolors, monotypes, drawings, and lithographs took place all over Italy. He was known particularly for his use of color, his portraits, and his impasto landscapes, which, according to the art critic Howard Devree, exhibited a "strange swirling strength" (*New York Times*, May 18, 1947). Levi once remarked that his year of exile in the south was an important influence on his painting, even more so than the war. In addition to painting and writing, he was so well known and trusted in the arts that he was appointed president of the Commission for the Reconstruction of the Province of Florence.

His autobiographical novel *The Watch* tells of life in several parts of Italy in the immediate postwar years. In typical Carlo Levi prose, he describes in brief but revealing sketches the people he meets, from authoritative government officials to peasants and the impoverished. The pages describing his automobile trip to Naples to visit his dying uncle make a grand short story: a group of unacquainted travelers and their luggage are thrown together for a journey and complete it despite failing tires and engines, long delays, and even a brigand at the side of the road. Chaucer would have happily told the tale.

The Linden Trees (*La Doppia Notte dei Tiggli*), a travel narrative of his visit to postwar Germany, was published in 1959. Most of the people he met there were artists and others involved in the humanities —that is, people much like him. He did not meet former Nazis, and therefore missed the opportunity to explore the thinking of that group. He spent much of his time in art museums, offering insightful comments on the works. Levi the rebel could not resist one slightly uncivilized act when, while crossing from East to West Germany, he came across the ruins of Göring's once palatial house. He tells of entering through a gaping hole in the wall, and, concealed from onlookers, "without thinking twice I took advantage of my momentary isolation to urinate . . . against the wall."

In Germany, with a bit of unintended irony, a former German soldier told Levi: "I've seen cathedrals, many beautiful ones, when I was in Italy. I was there during the war . . . the Italians are hospitable." But for Levi, with his strong political views, fascist Italy had been anything but hospitable.

Summing up his trip to a divided Germany, he reached back to his abandoned medical training for a metaphor: "This land which is in the heart of Europe, itself shaped like a heart, and which, swollen with obscure sentiments concealed beneath the protective armor of its breast, stubbornly beats to the rhythm of its machines. It has two ventricles, a right and a left, which do not alternate and do not know each other. Its valves are perfect, its heartbeats regular and sound. Everything is in place; everything has been miraculously restored." But, he added, "I felt there was a dark silence beneath the regular, mechanical beating of that great organ, a hollow silence made up of questions and terror. That heart, that mighty heart, that mysterious heart, was an empty heart."

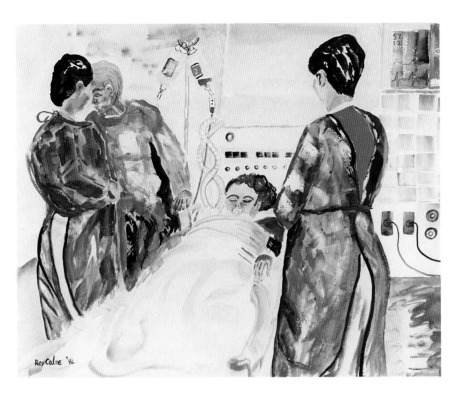

1. Sir Roy Calne, *The Operation*

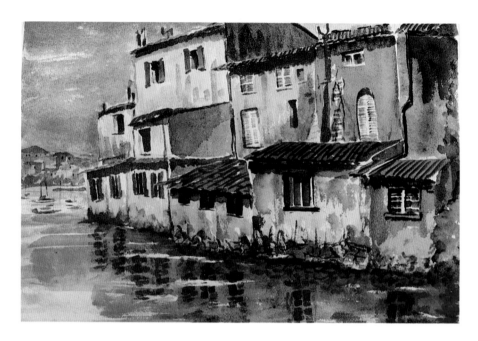

2. Ernest Craige, *Le Miroir*

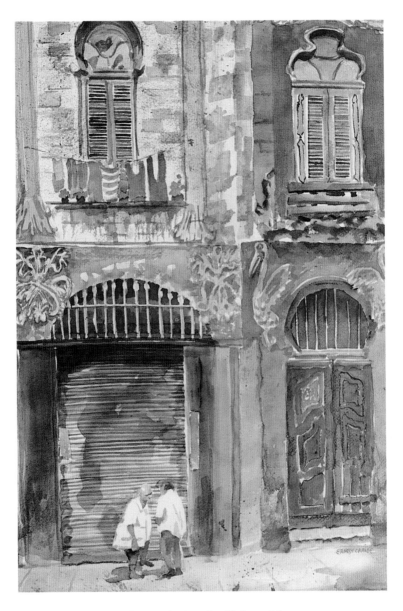

3. Ernest Craige, *La Habana Vieja*

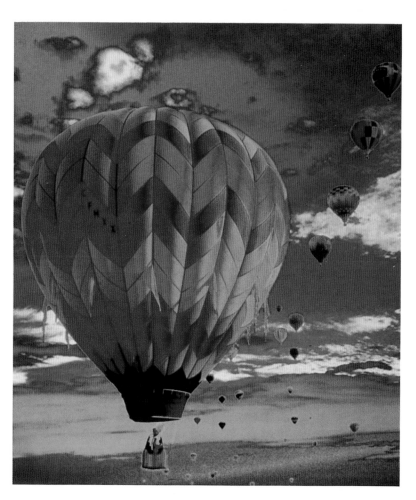

4. Mark Swartz, *To Fly*

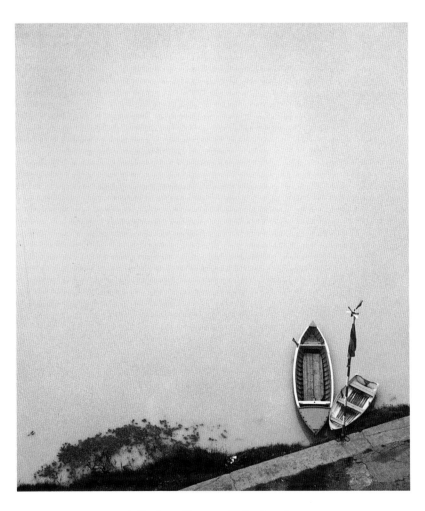

5. Barbara Young, *Uffizi Landing*

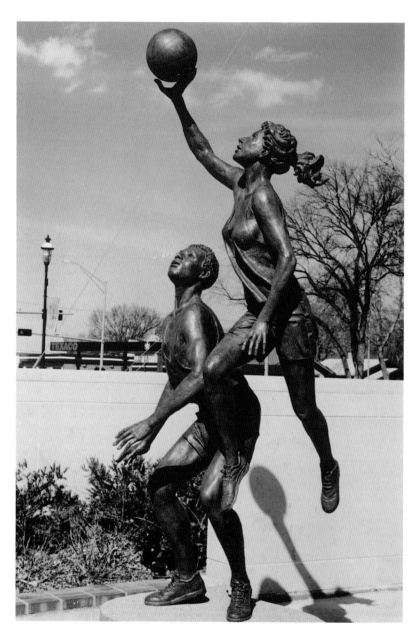

6. Wayne Southwick, *An American Dream*

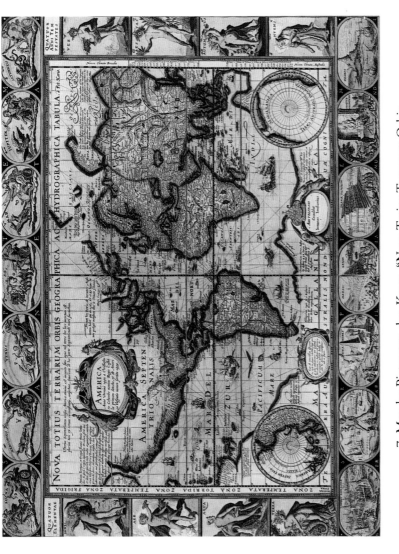

7. Map by Pieter van den Keere, "Nova Totius Terrarum Orbis Geographica Ac Hydrographica Tabula," 1608, from the collection of Harold Osher

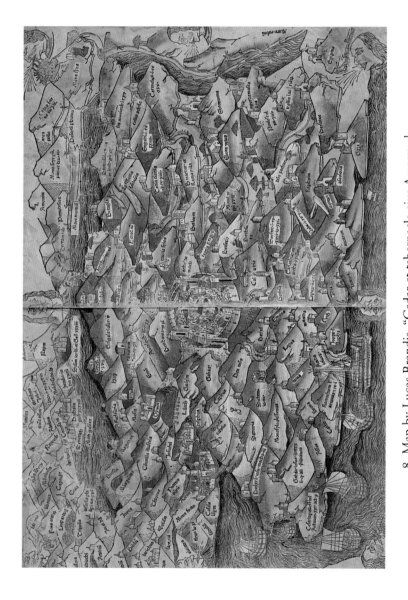

8. Map by Lucas Brandis, "Cedar et tabernacla eius Aras wecha unde baldach in Job," 1475, from the collection of Harold Osher

Carlo Levi's reluctance to practice medicine arises again in his writing when, in *Words Are Stones,* the narrative of a trip to Sicily, he writes, "We went . . . into all the houses and everywhere we encountered the most elementary problems of a world slavishly confined within the limits set by hunger and disease; and once again, as many years before, I was forced against my will to recall old and almost forgotten notions of medicine. In Spine Sante the answer to the offense of the outside world is not banditry but—feebler and more painful—disease and madness."

He describes madness in prose that modern-day textbooks might seek to emulate. "There was a young man sitting motionless in a chair: his old mother showed him to us and tried in vain to rouse him to speech: his apathetic schizophrenic silence had lasted for years. In a doorway stood another young man, thin faced, dim-eyed, his arms dangling at his sides—quite quiet at the moment, but his neighbors told us, when attacked by hunger, a raging madman."

Levi was a close friend of the Triestine poet, story writer, and antiquarian Umberto Saba (the pseudonym of Umberto Poli). Saba suffered persecution by the fascists because he was Jewish and, like many others, hid in Florence during that period. He wrote remarkable stories of the Jewish ghetto in Trieste and sent them to Levi, with the request that they not be published. Levi not only persuaded him to do otherwise but wrote the introduction to the book as well. Thanks to the brilliant translation of Estelle Gilson, "Gil Ebrei" ("The Jews") and other stories are available in English.

Painting occupied Levi wherever he was—confined, imprisoned, exiled, or in hiding. During such arduous times he produced, among other works, *Disegni dal Carcere* (1934) and *Dipinti del Confino* (1936). On one occasion the authorities coming to arrest him waited for him to finish a painting before leading him away.

Despite his treatment by the fascists, Levi emerged from his wartime hiding still loving Italy, its history, and its rich daily life. In *Eternal Italy,* he celebrated his remarkable homeland: "There is a little of everything in this all-embracing land, where nothing has perished, where the centuries are piled up, one on top of another, where pagan and Christian, prehistoric, classical, medieval and modern happily overlap. Every object is a recapitulation of what has gone before, and all contradictions seem to be lost in identity." The contadini were never far from his thoughts. In his exile among them he saw and felt the nature of their brutish existence. In the same volume, he wrote:

> In this silent world, bypassed by the pageant of history, where time seems to have come to a stop, there live the people to whom Italy owes its permanence and grandeur. Their ancient, highly original civilization, repeatedly subjugated but stubbornly and patiently surviving, is rich in human values; it is bound up with eternal realities, with the land and the seasons and the animals. Only love can provide a key to understanding its apparently impenetrable complexities. In this peasant world animals partake of the nature of angels and brothers. They live in the single-room house, and the family goes to sleep to the sound of a cow chewing its cud or a mule shuffling its feet. Men and their wives ride donkeys to their work every morning and back home at night, in a rhythm like that of a wave rolling to and from the shore.

The fall of fascism and the end of the war found Levi among Italy's prominent intellectuals. In 1945 he moved back to Rome and maintained a studio in a fashionable section. Entering politics as an independent, he was elected a senator in 1963 on a ticket backed by the Communist Party; he served two terms but was not reelected in 1972. The eternal intra- and interideological squabbles of the parties of the Left probably contributed to his defeat. The Italian Action Party, which he had helped form years earlier, had become hopelessly splintered.

In 1975, following his death from pneumonia, the *New York Times* obituary described a bon vivant popular among artists and creative persons as well as a local character easily recognized by taxi drivers and police. Long hair, flowery shirts, and gaudy suits were his style. In Rome, far removed in spirit and geography from his exile, he was "often the center of animated discussions at restaurant tables or on cafe terraces in the *Piazza del Popolo,* near his home until the wee hours." The Fondazione Carlo Levi in Rome and the Carlo Levi Museum, which occupies his house in Gagliano, help keep his memory alive.

We can't know if Carlo Levi would have been a good physician had he not abandoned medicine. He had the human traits necessary to respect his patients and work in their behalf, but the lure of painting and writing might have kept him from remaining scientifically up-to-date and technically adept. We can be assured, however, that he served his beloved Italy through his antifascism and through his painting and writing, which call the world's attention to the wretched human condition of a remote Italian village.

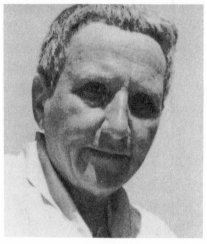

Like Carlo Levi, GERTRUDE STEIN (1874–
1946) is a well-known figure. Gerald Weissmann's
account of Stein's early years brings life to her
experiences. Unlike our other doctors afield, however,
Stein did not graduate from medical school, even
though she completed most requirements. This
medical background, coupled with her work at Woods
Hole in the Marine Biological Laboratory, makes her
a fitting addition to this book.

Gertrude Stein
and the Ctenophore

Gerald Weissmann, M.D.

The photograph shows a score of students in the summer dress of a century ago, collecting specimens at low tide from a harbor near Woods Hole, in Falmouth, Massachusetts. The harbor is Quissett, whose waters today remain rich in marine life. Its heights are still dominated by a Yankee cottage called "Petrel's Rest," with its familiar veranda and flagpole. The young people pictured are on a collecting trip for the course in invertebrate zoology at the Marine Biology Laboratory. The photo was taken on July 31, 1897: the young woman in the middle is Gertrude Stein. She has turned and is smiling at her brother Leo, who holds up a specimen jar: "Look what I've found!" he gestures to the photographer. Many in the group are also smiling; it is the height of summer, and they have disembarked at a marine Cythera where lush creatures drift on tides warmed by the Gulf Stream. Leo Stein has snared a ctenophore, a solitary, free-swimming member of the *hydromedusae:* a stunning trophy from the sea.

Gertrude Stein was twenty-three that summer; she had just finished Radcliffe and was to enter the Johns Hopkins Medical School in the fall. Having enrolled in the embryology course of the Marine Biology Laboratory, Gertrude often accompanied Leo and the invertebrate zoologists on collecting trips. She was on her way to becoming almost, but not quite, a doctor. In 1955, W. C. Curtis, who stands just to the right of Stein in white cap

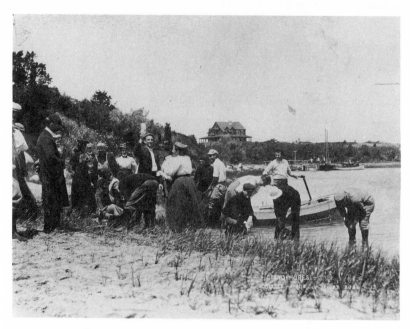

Gertrude Stein (center) facing her brother Leo,
Woods Hole, Massachusetts, 1897

and knee boots, remembered in the *Falmouth Enterprise:* "For us that
summer she was just a big fat girl waddling around the laboratory
and hoisting herself in and out of the row-boats on collecting trips."
He might have added that at the time she was still in thrall to her
fast-talking brother: some might read the photo as a record of a very
intense bond. Stein has written that as children she and Leo had
tramped alone in the woods of northern California; her adoring gaze
in that photo from Woods Hole suggests an American future for
them both—from the redwood forests to the Gulf Stream waters, as
it were.

But the photo suggests motifs other than those of a family ro-
mance; the image alone is a stunning icon of natural science. The
photo leads our eye, via the sight lines of Gertrude and another
young woman, straight to Leo, who looks to the lens with his prize
held high. Looking at the photo a century later, we know that the
scales of discovery tipped toward the sister, and we therefore tend to
read the picture as an action shot of the artist as a young woman.

There, on the beach at Quissett, at the dawn of a century whose art she will help form, she looks forever happy by a summer sea.

The picture also evokes memories of darker days in the middle of the twentieth century. The solitary, shimmering ctenophore, trapped in a jar, recalls aspects of Gertrude Stein other than her art. In Wendy Steiner's *Exact Resemblance to Exact Resemblance: The Literary Portraiture of Gertrude Stein* (1978), Frederick Dupee characterized her as "at once female and male, Jew and non-Jew, American *pur sang* and European peasant, artist and public figure." Catharine Stimpson asks her Rutgers students more bluntly: How did two Jewish lesbians survive the Nazis in France? As we've learned from a recent volume of Stein's letters, she and her companion, Alice B. Toklas, were by no means trapped by the war but voluntarily sat out the German Occupation in a French alpine resort. In line with her modernist infatuation with fascist politics in general, and her support of Franco's rebellion in particular, she spent the war years translating a collection of Marshal Pétain's speeches for an American audience, praising the Nazi puppet as the "George Washington" of France. Be that as it may, between the beach at Quissett and the 1940s in Culoz, she changed forever the way we read the English language.

No other picture of the young Stein shows her quite as perky as on that day at Quissett. In a group photo of her embryology class, taken later in the summer, she is preoccupied and unsmiling. Indeed, nothing about science or medicine seems to have given her much joy after her tussle with ctenophores. After indifferent attention to laboratory and clinic, she failed to graduate from the Johns Hopkins Medical School with her class of 1901. Although she had completed the bulk of her work, she seemed to have floundered over obstetrics —she who had gotten all that marine embryology right. She tells us that it was in the course of her obstetrical work that she became "aware of the Negroes" in the Baltimore clinics served by Johns Hopkins; from that experience emerged the story of Melanctha in *Three Lives* (1908). The mulatto abandons a humdrum doctor in favor of more louche companionship. To hear her tell it, Gertrude Stein and Johns Hopkins separated as if by mutual consent. In *The Autobiography of Alice B. Toklas* (1933), she relates: "The Professor who had flunked her asked her to come to see him. She did. He said, of course,

Miss Stein all you have to do is to take a summer course here and in the fall naturally you will take your degree. But not at all, said Gertrude Stein, you have no idea how grateful I am to you. I have so much inertia and so little initiative that very possibly if you had not kept me from taking my degree I would have, well, not taken to the practice of medicine, but at any rate to pathological psychology and you don't know how little I like pathological psychology, and how *all medicine bores me.* The professor was completely taken aback and that was the end of the Medical education of Gertrude Stein" (emphasis added).

Well, not exactly. Stein failed not pathological psychology but obstetrics. Moreover, her life at the Johns Hopkins of William Osler—who defined female medical students as "the third sex"—may have been many things, but it could not have been boring. The minutes of the Medical Faculty Advisory Board record that "the Dean presented the marks of the Graduating Class and on motion of Dr. Osler it was voted that Miss Gertrude Stein be not recommended for the degree of Doctor of Medicine." Whether from boredom with medicine or deeper battles of the self, no joy is evident in her 1901 class picture at Hopkins. She stands glumly, half-hidden in the back row behind other women and the shorter, swarthier of the men.

Later, in 1901, she left for Europe and, after aimless wanderings with her brother, settled in Paris to find her vocation. Gertrude soon outdistanced Leo, who had stopped dabbling in biology; she discovered new art and new friends on the banks of the Seine. By the time Picasso painted her in 1906, her Iberian portrait showed the confident young writer who was crafting *Three Lives* in the course of becoming—in the words of Carl Van Vechten—midwife to the twentieth century.

Those who look to details of biography for explanations of literary or artistic styles can usually extract as much material as needed to convince. Stein was born on the north side of Pittsburgh in 1874 to a prosperous German-Jewish clothing merchant; the family business was dissolved the year of her birth. Her father took the Stein family abroad for years of continental wandering and early education before returning to the United States and settling in Oakland, where a new family cable business was established. Although orphaned in adolescence, Stein was assured of an independent income for life; many of her American connections, first in San Francisco and then in Baltimore, were also the kin of wealthy textile merchants.

Stein's haut bourgeois, international background, which she shared with Henry James, has prompted Dupee and others to call attention to the mandarin elements her work shares with the Master. But it was Henry's brother, William (M.D., Harvard, 1869), who seems to have played a greater role in Stein's career. The most provocative explanation of how her unique style developed—its ontogeny as it were—was offered by B. F. Skinner, writing in the *Atlantic* of April 1935. In an article entitled "Has Gertrude Stein a Secret?" the Harvard professor of psychology traced Stein's technique to her undergraduate research work on automatic writing with William James, Skinner's predecessor as professor of experimental psychology at Harvard. The case is persuasive, even if Skinner's aesthetic verdict on Stein's later work is a tad harsh. But another influence, that of Jacques Loeb, her instructor at Woods Hole, has not escaped notice. In the formative years of her compositional style, Gertrude Stein owned that she was an old-fashioned mechanist, a reductionist of the school of Jacques Loeb. Her revolution of words owed as much to Loeb's *The Mechanistic Conception of Life* (1912) as to her study "Normal Motor Automatism," which she had written for William James, or to the *Demoiselles d'Avignon* (1907) of her Picasso years.

When Stein trod the beach at Quissett, Jacques Loeb (1859–1924) was the leader of a new, mechanistic school of American biology that tried to explain biological phenomena through physics. In 1897, Loeb was teaching the physiology course at Woods Hole, and the implications of his biophysical approach were the talk of the Marine Biology Lab. He had demonstrated that the chemical nature of salts in the environment of a cell controlled its irritability, movement, and reproduction in predictable ways. He was on his way to creating life in a dish, to forming fatherless sea urchins by chemical means. Parthenogenesis was announced two years later, but his work on tropisms and salt solutions had already paved the way for what Loeb termed, in *The Mechanistic Conception,* the fundamental task of physiology: "to determine whether or not we shall be able to produce living matter artificially."

Stein had heard the siren song of vital forces from the voice of gentle William James; and she had worked with one of Loeb's mechanist friends, Franklin Pierce Mall, in the embryology course at Woods Hole and at Johns Hopkins. But by the time she published *Three Lives,* her critics got it just right: she was on the side of the mechanists. In Steiner's *Exact Resemblance,* Wyndham Lewis—another modernist fan of fascism—argued in his review that Stein's book put demotic speech into the "metre of an obsessing time" and, although "undoubtably intended as an epic contribution to the present mass-democracy," gave "to the life it patronizes the mechanical bias of its creator."

The careers of Stein and Loeb ran somewhat in parallel. Orphaned in youth, both were brought up by well-off relatives as secular Jews, Stein in California and Loeb in the Rhineland. Both emigrated as young adults; both spoke their adopted languages with awkward accents. Early in their careers, both performed experiments on brain function that caught the attention of William James; Loeb had written to James in search of a faculty position in the New World. When Stein entered Hopkins, she worked on mechanical models of spinal tracts with Mall, Loeb's colleague from Woods Hole and the University of Chicago. Both Stein and Loeb engaged the far-from-casual interest of B. F. Skinner, who was persuaded by Loeb's argument in *The Organism as a Whole* (1916) that mechanist principles could be applied to the study and control of behavior. Skinner was a true believer in Loeb's *Mechanistic Conception of Life,* and it surprised no one that when he turned his attention to Stein, he deciphered her work in the language of nerves.

Skinner was the first to draw attention to Stein's undergraduate work on automatic writing. He pointed out the origins of her verbal experiments by unearthing a paper entitled "Normal Motor Automatism," published in the *Psychological Review* of September 1896 by Leon M. Solomons and Gertrude Stein, reflecting their work with the Harvard psychological laboratory (with William James as their professor). Solomons and Stein reported on experiments designed to test whether a second personality—as displayed in cases of hysteria —could be called forth deliberately from normal subjects. The two authors undertook to see how far they could "split" their personality by eliciting automatic writing under a variety of test conditions. They concluded that hysteria is a *"disease* of the *attention"* (their italics), basing their argument on the finding that when distracted or inattentive, normal subjects show the abnormal motor behavior of hysterics.

Skinner showed little interest in Solomons and Stein's discussion of hysteria, being more concerned with tracing Stein's literary style to her experiences of automatic writing. Using themselves as test subjects, Solomons and Stein were able to show that with a little practice they could regularly produce automatic writing as they took dictation while reading another text: "The word is written or half-written before the subject knows anything about it, or perhaps he never knows anything about it. For overcoming this habit of attention we found constant repetition of one word of great value." After they had trained themselves by this sort of cognitive drill, and after sessions with ouija boards to call up their alter egos, automatic writing became easy. Stein found it convenient to read what her arm wrote, following three or four words behind her pencil. In this fashion, "a phrase would seem to get into the head and keep repeating itself at every opportunity, and hang over from day to day even. The stuff written was grammatical, and the words and phrases fitted together all right, but there was not much connected thought."

Skinner—a traditionalist with respect to the arts—argued that these experiments explained why there appeared to be two Gertrude Steins. The first Stein was accessible and had written such serious works as *Three Lives* and the *Autobiography of Alice B. Toklas;* the second Stein was dense and wrote stuff that had words and phrases fitted together all right but without connected thought. This other Stein had written *Tender Buttons* (1915), her portraits, and *The Making of Americans* (1925). *Four Saints in Three Acts* (1934) was yet to come! Skinner gave mild positive reinforcement to the first Stein, but strong negative reinforcement to the second, chiding her that "the mere generation of the effects of repetition and surprise is not in itself a literary achievement." Skinner complained that the second Stein gives no clue as to the personal history or cultural background of the author and dismissed her most adventurous book with a phrase from their common master, William James: *"Tender Buttons* is the stream of consciousness of a woman without a past." It is, of course, next to *Q.E.D.*, her most homoerotic work; no past, indeed!

Skinner's theory of the two Steins permitted him to "dismiss one part of Gertrude Stein's writing as a probably ill-advised experiment and to enjoy the other and very great part without puzzlement." The irony seemed to have been lost on our leading reductionist that he was reducing Stein's new style to its most arid origin: the knack of automatic writing she had acquired in the course of her undergraduate experiments.

Other interpretations might occur to those who believe that behavior—not to speak of literature—might be described in more complex, dynamic ways. William James wrote Stein to acknowledge his receipt of *Three Lives:* "I promise you that it shall be read some time! You see what a swine I am to have pearls cast before him! As a rule reading fiction is as hard to me as trying to hit a target by hurling feathers at it. I need *resistance,* to cerebrate!" What a challenge to fiction by the brother of Henry James! But, of course, Gertrude Stein had not simply written yet another work of fiction; she had in fact fabricated a new language. Stein's language turned the quiet elisions of homoerotic love into a seamless web of modern prose. No wonder she encountered enough resistance for a gaggle of Jameses.

Her incantation to the Liberation—"What a day is today that is what a day it was day before yesterday, what a day!"—is not only pure Stein but can also be read as an utterance of disguise (*Selected Writings*). In either case, it is couched in the language of our century: short repetitive sequences. Such sequences run through modern literature from Christian Morgenstern to Kurt Vonnegut, from Samuel Beckett to Harold Pinter; they charge the beat of modern music from rock to Philip Glass. Short repetitive sequences also constitute the language of our genes; when we talk DNA or RNA, we speak pure Stein. We would not be surprised to hear a molecular biologist explaining a stretch of DNA in the one-letter code of nucleic acids: What a TAA is ATAA that is ATA what a TAA it was, what a TATAA, what a TAA, what a TATAA!

But Stein's story, which began with Loeb and the ctenophore at Quissett, ends on a note that reverts to a murkier mood of William

James. In his *Essays on Faith, Ethics, and Morals* (1887), James—who found the Civil War too rich for his blood—had assured the Unitarians that "[I] myself have little fear for our Anglo-Saxon race. Its moral, aesthetic, and practical wants form too dense a stubble to be mown down by any scientific Occam's razor that has yet been forged. The knights of the razor will never form among us more than a sect."

Gertrude Stein and Alice Toklas, along with their servants, sat out the grimmer stages of Hitler's war in a villa in Culoz, a French town about thirty miles from the Swiss border. They appear to have been protected from the roundup of Jews and foreigners by the prominent French fascist Bernard Faÿ, who served Pétain and his puppet government as director of the Bibliothèque Nationale. Faÿ also edited the monthly *Les Documents Maçonniques,* which was devoted to rooting out freemasonry or belief in "exclusive scientifism," as James would have it. From July 1940 until June 1944, Faÿ was also an editor of the only journal financed by the Germans, the anti-Jewish *La Gerbe.* Tried and convicted as a war criminal, he nevertheless obtained for Stein and Toklas letters of support during the immediate postwar period; he also took care of their art collection during their stay in the Alps. Evidence has recently come forth that Stein was no unwilling "victim" of the Nazis; she undertook to introduce a collection of Pétain's speeches with this outrageous comparison: "We did not understand defeat enough to sympathize with the french people and with their Maréchal Pétain, who like George Washington, and he is very like George Washington because he too is first in war first in peace and first in the hearts of his countrymen, who like George Washington has given them courage in their darkest moment held them together through their times of desperation and has always told them the truth and in telling them the truth has made them realize that the truth would set them free." Perhaps the worst untruth she perpetuated, published in Edward M. Burns and Ulla E. Dydo's *Letters of Gertrude Stein and Thornton Wilder* (1996), was her bland assurance that the French were all darlings throughout the war:

> Speaking of all this there is this about a Jewish woman, a
> Parisienne, well known in the Paris world. She and her fam-

ily took refuge in Chambéry [a stone's throw from Culoz and the town where Stein and Toklas shopped each Tuesday] when the persecutions against the Jews began in Paris. And then later, when there was no southern zone, all the Jews were supposed to have the fact put on their carte d'identité and their food card, she went to the prefecture to do so and the official whom she saw looked at her severely Madame he said, have you any proof with you that you are a Jewess, why no she said, well he said if you have no actual proof that you are a Jewess, why do you come and bother me, why she said I beg your pardon, no he said I am not interested unless you can prove you are a Jewess, good day he said and she left. It was she who told the story. Most of the French officials were like that really like that.

Well, not exactly. Within a few blocks of M. Faÿ's office at the Bibliothèque, French officials rounded up hundreds of French "Jewesses" and their children to pack them off in cattle cars. "N'oubliez pas!" the stone tablet reads today at the Marché des Blanc-Manteaux. Many of Stein's coterie turned their backs on these events, while not a few were Pétain sympathizers or worse. It is no accident that in *Axel's Castle,* Edmund Wilson ranks Stein with W. B. Yeats, Ezra Pound, T. S. Eliot, and Paul Valéry. Like Stein, the doyens of prewar modernism linked a taste for avant-garde literature with one for *arrière-garde* politics. Again like Stein, many of the French modernists— from Cocteau to Gide, Péguy to Claudel, Lartigue to Maillot, even Picasso to Matisse—behaved during the Nazi Occupation as if the struggles of our time were simply an unpleasant interruption to their life in art. It may also not have been an accident that when Gertrude Stein was asked about the bomb that ended the war against Japan, she replied: "They asked me what I thought of the atomic bomb. I said I had not been able to take any interest in it" (*Selected Writings*).

Perhaps such attitudes as boredom with medicine or disinterest in nuclear weapons are the high price some artists pay to gladden their muse. Or perhaps the strict homophobia of William Osler and the late Victorians has much to answer for. Whatever. In the light of her undoubted genius, the tribute Stein paid to Picasso, in her *Picasso*

(1938), can be read as her own ambiguous lesson of self-love and hate: "A creator is contemporary, he understands what is contemporary when the contemporaries do not yet know it, but he is contemporary and as the twentieth century is a century which sees the earth as no one has ever seen it, the earth has a splendor that it never had, and as everything destroys itself in the twentieth century and nothing continues, so then the twentieth century has a splendor which is its own and of this century, [it has] that strange quality of an earth that one has never seen and of things destroyed as they have never been destroyed as they have never been destroyed."

Part 4

Astronautics

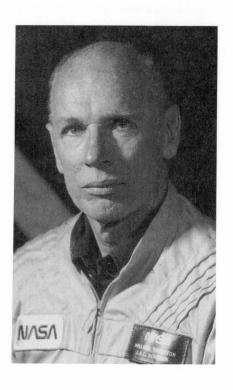

Building on an early fascination with science and technology, WILLIAM THORNTON managed to combine an extraordinary proficiency in physics and engineering with medicine and physiology. His love of flying, together with his skills as a medical scientist, led him in 1963 to join the National Aeronautics and Space Administration space program as a scientist-astronaut. His unique experiences in the *Challenger* spacecraft include being the first doctor to perform a physical examination in space. He has certainly reached the greatest height of any of our contributors.

The Sky's No Limit

William Thornton, M.D.

Faison, North Carolina, was a good place to grow up, especially during the Depression. My father took time to tramp the woods with me, teach me manual skills, and transmit his sense of wonder at natural and constructed phenomena; my mother epitomized personal industry. I was eleven years old when my father died and serious work began; I delivered newspapers, worked as a manual laborer and a theater projectionist and, finally, opened my own radio shop. From earliest childhood I loved airplanes; I could never hear a plane go by without looking up at the sky (and still can't). My other great passion was science, especially as it pertained to the human body and, increasingly, physics.

In spite of an aversion to the rigors of mathematics, I enrolled as a physics major at the University of North Carolina (UNC). Instead of pursuing scholarships, I hitchhiked home every weekend to make money in my radio and television shop, tried out for football and survived four years as the only amateur member of a nationally ranked team, and joined the Air Force ROTC on the premise that another war was inevitable. That decision cost me an extra year of school, but it paid a stipend.

During the Korean War, I spent three years at the Air Proving Ground in Florida developing systems to test and augment new air force interceptors. A temporary assignment as a decontamination officer for bacteriological weaponry reawakened my interest in medicine, so I reluctantly dropped my long-held plans for flight school.

My success with military electronics persuaded me that

similar technology could be applied to medicine. But after working briefly at the North Carolina Memorial Hospital (NCMH), I realized that I needed a medical education to make this sort of work useful. Medical school was obviously going to require time and money —hence my move to join Del Mar Engineering, a small aircraft company in Los Angeles that was interested in producing some of my air force inventions.

Finally, in 1959, by which time I had married and begun a family, I returned to UNC. Moving from moneyed management to first-year medical student was a step down in several ways.

I had surmised correctly that medicine was lagging behind by decades in the use of the available technology, but this situation was about to change drastically. The electrocardiogram (EKG), for example, was limited to a few heartbeats recorded on paper tape from a patient lying as quietly as possible. But the EKG was urgently needed during surgical procedures and in many diagnostic situations as well. A high-frequency transistor had recently become available, making it possible for me to build a miniature EKG transmitter that patients could wear as needed. Soon every operating suite in NCMH was equipped with my little transmitters, which were monitored by commercial oscilloscopes—a first in the country and a forerunner of the anesthesia monitoring now required by law. As expected, morbidity dropped sharply. Application of such technology to cardiology became my next goal, to be followed by physiology and neurology.

Just before my graduation from medical school in 1963, at the age of thirty-four, I attended a symposium at San Antonio's School of Aerospace Medicine (SAM), where reports on recent space flights renewed my dreams not only of flying but of flying in space. The age limit set by the National Aeronautics and Space Administration (NASA) disqualified me as an astronaut, but the air force also had a more or less secret manned space program. After some quiet negotiations and a return to active duty, I headed to San Antonio. My justification for leaving traditional medicine was that my unique background could produce developments in space medicine that could have untold benefits on earth. This is now NASA's mantra, especially at budget time.

In some ways my year of air force internship was idyllic, especially for the family. When evacuation flights from Vietnam and other parts of the world landed, the work was grueling; but I had time off, along with regular pay, so there was no need to build EKG transmitters on the kitchen table in order to keep food on it. In addition, San Antonio, like several other old Spanish towns in America, proved fascinating.

At the end of that satisfying year, I joined the Brooks Air Force Base Aerospace Medical Division, as planned. With Colonel Jack Ord, I was to develop a medical investigation program for the Manned Orbiting Laboratory (MOL), the space effort of the United States Air Force.

After completing the flight surgeons' short course at SAM, I pinned on my first set of wings and began to fly again, first taking care of critical patients on "Air Evac" flights and then testing my developments in zero-gravity (or zero-G) flights. Still on duty at Brooks Air Force Base were many well-known American and German figures from aviation history. The superb instrument shop was staffed by some of the Luftwaffe's best machinists and a number of do-anything Texans. Thanks to their skills and eighteen months of unceasing development, I was able to build the first successful mass-measurement devices for space and several other instruments for the MOL. Weightlessness makes weighing impossible, yet mass measurement was essential to sorting out such problems as the crews' initial rapid loss of weight in flight and their hypotension, dizziness, tachycardia, and occasional fainting after flight. Once the word was out, we also developed both small and body (human-scale) mass-measurement devices to support several NASA *Skylab* projects. But neither the USAF space program nor my personal aspiration to fly in space was progressing well.

Before resigning myself to medicine on earth, I made one last effort to get into NASA's program—just as another scientist-astronaut program was announced, this one with a higher age limit. The next six months were spent on an emotional roller coaster with two thousand other semifinalists, then two hundred finalists. At long last, Alan Shepherd, then chief astronaut officer of the Johnson Space Center (JSC), called and asked, "Do you want to come aboard?"

After a few weeks, however, the chief of flight operations urged our class of scientist-astronauts to resign: two of the three *Skylabs* had been canceled, and we were neither needed nor wanted. But all of us would have robbed banks to stay, and none of our Excess Eleven (XS 11) class left until a couple were washed out in flying school. As a student pilot older than many first-line jet pilots being removed for reasons of age, I came under special scrutiny by USAF generals—who also underestimated the power of obsession. Finally my pilot wings were pinned on.

Skylab was the world's first space station, cobbled from *Apollo* hardware under budget restraints. Both NASA and its contractors needed the most realistic possible testing of medical procedures and hardware on *Skylab*, as there would be no spares aboard and no way to send up replacements. Two colleagues and I volunteered for the Skylab Medical Experiments Altitude Test, a thankless job of living under the rigors of a fifty-six-day space mission and shaking down simulated procedures and equipment while locked in a sixteen-foot chamber that was going nowhere. Preparation for the "mission" included collecting all our body wastes wherever we went and eating only two thousand calories a day of freeze-dried food, plus sugar cookies and lemon drops "as necessary." After the six weeks of base-line data collection, we kissed our wives good-bye, prebreathed pure oxygen to avoid the bends, and paraded past the news media into our closed world of steel and aluminum. Fifty-six days later we marched out of the longest chamber test on record, having demonstrated that key hardware items would cripple *Skylab* if taken along in their present state. The expensive and elaborate space urinal had failed seven times; and the cycle ergometer (essential to several studies and the only exercise equipment aboard) had failed twice. Numerous smaller glitches also occurred.

NASA still had the technical and administrative capacity to fix things, and quickly. At great cost, a simple new system for urine collection was built; the ergometer bearings were properly installed; many other hardware and procedural changes were made; and contingency food was added. Eight months later, the last of Wernher Von Braun's American-German Saturn Vs shook Cape Canaveral (now Cape Kennedy) for miles around and lifted the 150,000-pound *Skylab I* laboratory into orbit. But doom and gloom soon set in: insulation and one solar panel had torn off during *Skylab's* ascent, and its other major solar panel was jammed. The lab's contents were roasting in space. Again NASA ingenuity saved a mission: in the course of ten hectic days a giant parasol had been constructed.

Skylab II was launched uneventfully, and its crew used heavy-duty tools to cut away debris and free the jammed solar panel on *Skylab I*. They deployed the parasol through a space port over the overheated craft and, as the lab cooled, began the first of three missions that to this day are scientific landmarks in space.

After twenty-eight days, *Skylab II* returned and a few days later *Skylab III* was launched, heavily laden with last-minute equipment, including my gear for arm-strength exercise. The second crew not only performed all planned experiments but found time for extra studies, returning fifty-six days later from the longest, most productive mission to date—but barely able to walk.

Skylab IV went up full of replacement items and ad hoc experiments, including a locomotor exercise device dubbed "Thornton's Revenge" by the crew. The third crew's new record of eighty-four days in orbit generated unprecedented amounts of data, and the men boarded the recovery ship almost jauntily in the best physical condition of any *Skylab* crew. During these three missions I communicated with the crew in flight on one shift and then regularly worked another shift, at first on the mass of new human data from space but increasingly on the creation of additional experiments and equipment, especially for exercise. *Skylab's* solar, ultraviolet, radiation, and earth observatories and its technical studies (involving three mass-measurement devices) produced mountains of data. *Skylab* also produced a comprehensive view of the human body's beautiful adaptation to the totally new environment of weightlessness. Although this adaptation left the body unable to function normally on return to earth, or on other bodies with strong gravity, *Skylab* had shown that essential functions, such as locomotion, could be preserved.

After the success of the *Apollo* missions in space travel and of *Skylab* in long-duration flight, NASA was poised for true interplanetary exploration. Instead, *Skylab,* larger and more efficient than the subsequent Russian *Mir,* was cast adrift. All human space-flight resources were devoted to a low-orbit transportation system, the space shuttle, scheduled to fly in 1978. Many astronauts left the program rather than wait for it, but six of the XS 11 hung on as the launch was delayed year after year. With NASA's approval, I repeated a year of clinical medicine, developed commercial medical instruments, and worked on shuttle problems, especially the difficulties humans experience in space.

Finally, in 1981, John Young and Bob Crippen flew the first shuttle. From a T-38 six miles above the launch, one watched a tiny white arrowhead on twin columns of smoke rise rapidly until, in a matter of seconds, it was lost in blue sky. After two days it reentered earth's atmosphere above the Indian Ocean, glided across the Pacific, and landed on California salt flats, its white sides seared by super-heated air during reentry.

The shuttle was a spectacular bird, but one with many problems —and, indeed, a fatal flaw. It also reemphasized human problems such as space motion sickness (SMS) and orthostasis, as well as transient weakness during and after landing. The news media raised a hue and cry over safety, an issue NASA could not ignore. The first planned investigation of SMS on *Spacelab I* was years away, and the shuttle had no room for currently available lab equipment. Because astronauts were able to make valid programmed neurological studies in orbit using miniature hardware, I proposed and quickly built a miniature neurophysiological lab for the shuttle. A series of neurological investigations was performed on shuttle flights four through seven, yielding an ever-increasing volume of data. Norm Thagard, M.D., had been added to Sally Ride's flight to conduct the now-extensive studies, and I was added to shuttle flight eight to use my hardware as I saw fit—a dream flight for me. The flight plan included launching a satellite for India, demonstrating the capacity of the shuttle's remote manipulator arm to remove and replace a dummy satellite from the payload bay, and other routine tasks. Unique aspects were a nighttime launch and landing and the presence of astronaut Guy Bluford, the first African American in space. Along with readying new instruments for studies in space, I underwent the usual extensive training in various simulators.

The local weather was questionable during the launch-readiness review, and at midnight thunderstorms continued to rage as we prepared for the flight. I donned the flight suit and instruments to record everything possible—blood pressure, heart rate, eye motion, and the like. We had the usual prelaunch breakfast, without the steak and eggs, and climbed aboard the crew bus amid lightning and the flashing of cameras. Three miles later, a lone guard waved us onto the eerily deserted launch pad.

We launched successfully, lighting up the cape for miles until, a few seconds later, we were in solid cloud. After waiting for sixteen years, at age fifty-four I was the oldest astronaut to fly; surrounded by visual target lights and instruments, I was determined to squeeze every possible bit of information out of each moment. For an experienced pilot it wasn't a rough ride; when the solids fell away after two minutes, the flight was as smooth as glass. G-loads built until they suddenly went to zero, with the familiar slight upward surge of weightlessness. Unlike my previous accumulated hours of weightlessness in zero-G aircraft, this persisted after thirty seconds and didn't go away for a week. My body had already begun to react, as blood rushed to my head from my legs. Although some had claimed disorientation at this point, my nervous system was not tumbling and my vision was normal.

After I had recorded my physiological responses with electrodes and pressure cuffs, I began to set up my lab. A quick neurological exam of a fellow astronaut showed nothing abnormal, until, with eyes closed, he was tilted forward and came up shouting, "Don't do that!" This incident convinced me that space-motion sickness was the product of erroneous signals from an inner-ear sensor that required weight to function normally. A short time later, without warning, we both had a brief, violent bout of emesis, followed by increasing lethargy, malaise, and anorexia, but without the nausea and sweating of motion sickness experienced on earth. SMS had arrived but suddenly and completely departed thirty-six hours later. During that time we continued working, unhappy but effective.

For the next week I lived on the mid-deck and in the airlock, where I slept about four hours a night, wedged between two space suits. Otherwise I pursued a dozen studies on myself and the crew, including the collection of my own blood and urine.

The ever-changing panorama visible from the flight deck was a

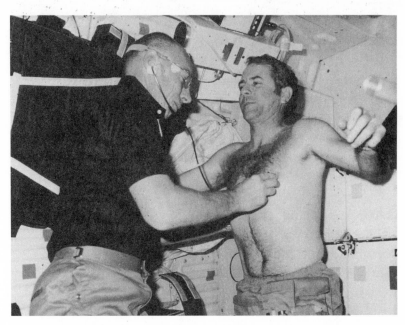

William Thornton performing the first physical exam in space

constant temptation to skip work. I managed to see sunrises and sunsets with indescribable depths of blue and gold every ninety minutes, night storms over Africa with lightning so intense that it illuminated our payload bay, and a few other unforgettable scenes. The daily round included communal meals of freeze-dried food, careful use of the high-tech waste-management system (notwithstanding its design flaws), and public relations events such as photos with various institutional banners and flags and a presidential news conference. My only regret was having to eat and sleep, because much was left unfinished.

When it came time to return to earth, we slowed *Challenger* enough to skim the top atmosphere and glided down for half an orbit around earth. During this brief period, a frenzy of studies took place, for our bodies began reversing their adaptation to weightlessness, our blood and fluids now draining from head to feet, among myriad other adjustments. No instruments were needed to show that some senses had made remarkable adjustments in orbit: when we felt we had reached 1G (normal weight), it turned out that we were pulling about one quarter of that load, and it felt a lot heavier as our craft slowed. At Edwards Air Force Base we fell out of the black night into blinding light in a scene that would have made Hollywood proud — and touched down so smoothly that I didn't know we were on the runway until lights flashed by. Our bodies knew we were back, for it took maximum effort to heave ourselves out of our seats and stagger around. Gaining strength by the minute, we still kept a firm grip on the rail as we came down the steps. The standard postflight medical exams, a 2:00 A.M. press conference, the flight back to Houston, and still more examinations followed before we finally were allowed to go to bed. Twelve hours later, it was take out the garbage, as usual.

Earthly demands ensued: to reduce and clarify data and to report them; to undergo debriefings; to fill requests for press releases, which ranged from the 21 Club to an uproarious barbecue in Faison's fire station. Experience plus experimental data had shown that the shuttle could be safely landed by human hands and that the dreaded SMS was no more than a transient nuisance. My medical practice resumed its deliberate pace, but to my surprise I soon received another flight assignment, to STS-51B, a medical-establishment flight.

NASA had made great investments in animal research, especially at Ames Research Center. I had participated in several mission simulations in which animals were a major part of the payload. These simulations tested only procedures, however, for flight hardware wasn't yet ready. Other preflight problems occurred on this first mixed mission, including demonstrations by animal-rights activists. The four simians trained for the flight were found to be carriers of monkey B virus, which can be fatal to humans, and were therefore replaced at the last minute by two others, one of whom was a lab pet. My goal was finally reduced to returning all forty-eight rats and two monkeys alive.

After liftoff, *Challenger* turned north to parallel the eastern coast of the United States. Two minutes later, Cape Fear slipped by. The nature of an entire flight can often be predicted in its first few hours. Even before we unstrapped, sounds of vomiting were heard, a hatch wouldn't open properly, and the power supply on a major experiment failed. It became the longest day of my life when, after searching an hour for a misstowed bag, I opened it and fifty unsecured medical sample tubes flew all over the lab. The next day, when the outer doors of the monkey cages were opened, a jet of crumbled food and waste flew into the lab, instead of the specified suction of cabin air into the cage. Duct tape saved the day—it seems unlikely that a space mission can ever be completed without it.

Another crisis involved the pet monkey who, unhappy with weightlessness and isolation, went on a hunger strike. Scientists on the ground insisted he was suffering SMS and would soon eat normally. On the fourth day, determined that we weren't going to bring back a dead monkey, I opened the door and began playing with him. In an hour he was feeding himself, voraciously. And, as on some previous missions, neither the space toilet nor the urine-measurement system worked properly.

In contrast, the physical science experiments, such as growing crystals and modeling the earth's atmosphere, were successful. During it all, we enjoyed glorious views—vast stretches of Siberia's green firs and white snow and hundreds of miles of shifting blue, green, and red curtains of the aurora borealis falling into the atmosphere at night. *Challenger* landed with all the animals very much alive, as planned.

My final chapter with the space program began on my return to Johnson Space Center. An immediate and crucial problem was the waste-management system, which threatened to abort longer shuttle missions with large crews. No problem was too sacrosanct or too basic for me to attack, and a prototype toilet was soon tested successfully in flight.

Ten months after our flight, the world was stunned by the news that the *Challenger* had blown up minutes after takeoff.

Three years later Americans gingerly went back into space, and a new management team was in place. I waited for the call to fix the problems that needed fixing, but NASA was no longer pushing human frontiers. Finally my strongest feature, my back, let me down and one of my most feared acquaintances, a wonderfully skilled neurosurgeon, irrevocably closed the field of high-performance aviation and space flight to me.

Hundreds of shelf feet of archives have documented my wandering, and the prototype space gymnasium I developed, along with other gear, is now in museums. Books still wait to be written, but for now I am trying to pass on to medical students and graduates what dedicated teachers such as Ernie Craige, my professor of cardiology at UNC, gave me.

There are still fields that do not require an intact spinal column, but they may be too distant for an old doctor. Then again, maybe not.

Part 5

The Spiritual Life

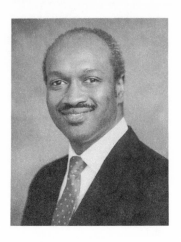

RAY HAMMOND, the son of a Baptist preacher
and a public schoolteacher, graduated in Near Eastern
Languages and Literature from Harvard in 1971, as
part of the first wave of black students admitted to
mostly white institutions. Since graduating from
Harvard Medical School, he has devoted his life to a
ministry of healing. After a surgical residency and
practice in emergency medicine, he studied religion
and was ordained in the African Methodist Episcopal
(A.M.E.) Church. In 1992, he became pastor of the
Bethel A.M.E. Church, which he founded. Beyond
healing his patients' bodies, he endeavors to treat the
human condition and to find new ways of reducing
urban violence.

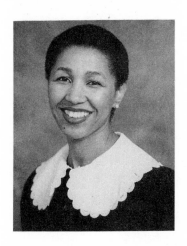

GLORIA WHITE-HAMMOND, the daughter of an air force sergeant and a homemaker, graduated from Tufts Medical School and later joined the South End Community Health Center in Boston. After marriage to Ray Hammond, she became an associate pastor at Bethel A.M.E. Church and graduated from Harvard Divinity School, while continuing to be active in pediatric and adolescent medicine. The Hammonds demonstrate how medicine and faith in God can be combined to heal the poor in health as well as the poor in spirit. The religious fervor they demonstrate in their efforts to remedy problems of the inner city reaches beyond their physical ministrations into their emotional and spiritual strengths. The Hammonds have lived an example of holistic medicine at its very best.

A Ministry of Healing

Ray A. Hammond, M.D., and
Gloria E. White-Hammond, M.D.,
with the assistance of Sheila Lennon

Ray A. Hammond, M.D.

Born and raised in Philadelphia, I am the son of a Baptist preacher and a schoolteacher. The words and deeds of both parents instilled in me a love for faith and knowledge. I was taught the old adage that service to others is the rent one pays for being on earth. My pursuit of faith was nurtured by song, sermon, and the search for truth in my own life and in the lives of others. My pursuit of knowledge was nurtured by a schoolteacher-mother who continues to study new subjects to this day and a preacher-father who died in his seventies while working on a master's degree. With this lineage, I entered Harvard College at age fifteen as a sophomore—part of the first wave of black students admitted to predominantly white institutions in the wake of the civil rights movement.

Those four college years were about as turbulent as any I have experienced. They were a time of student takeovers, protests against Vietnam, the winding down of the civil rights movement, the windup of black power, the death of Martin Luther King, Jr., Robert Kennedy, and God (at least according to some). Before it was over, I had questioned my emotional stability, my intellectual capability, my political beliefs, and my faith. But these were also years of rebirth. I learned some things about resilience, humility, and the tension between principles and pragmatism. I rediscovered my faith in God and my love for

Christ—not simply as the child of Christian parents but as a man who had learned to wrestle with this faith for himself. I graduated in 1971 with a major in Near Eastern Languages and Literature and a clear understanding that I would pursue the study of medicine. As I was so poignantly reminded by a friend and spiritual adviser named Cecilia Bryant, I would do fine as long as I remembered that I "was called not to a career in medicine but to a ministry of healing." Fulfilling that calling has been my aim ever since.

During medical school and residency, four significant events occurred. First, in 1973 I married my friend and life companion, Gloria White-Hammond, herself a medical student at Tufts University. Second, in 1976 I accepted a call to the ministry. Gloria and I assumed at the time that this would mean, among other things, that we would serve together as medical missionaries in a foreign country or in a medically underserved area in America. Little did we know that our mission work would be quite different. Third, from 1977 to 1982 Gloria and I became resident advisers at one of the Harvard undergraduate houses. There we became involved in campus ministry through the Seymour Society—a Christian fellowship dedicated to producing well-grounded Christians. We also became involved in an effort (then called the Efficacy Committee and now the Efficacy Institute) to boost the academic achievement of minority students in college and lower the dropout rates in inner-city high schools. This latter work played a pivotal role in our understanding of how one could bring healing not only to physical but to psychological and social problems as well. Finally, in 1979 and 1982 I became a father to two bright and beautiful daughters, Mariama and Adiya. Living with members of the next generation on a daily basis makes one's obligation to them remarkably clearer.

In 1981, I completed a surgical residency in the Harvard Fifth Surgical Service of the New England Deaconess Hospital, after which I began practicing emergency medicine full-time. Concurrently, I enrolled in the Harvard Graduate School of Arts and Sciences, where I obtained an M. A. in the Study of Religion in 1984. In 1982, I was ordained as an elder in the African Methodist Episcopal Church.

In my mind, the call to medicine and the ministry has seldom, if ever, conflicted. As I saw it, both came from the same source, and both, at their best, are committed to meeting some of the most basic human needs. I've been struck again and again by the fact that both medical practitioners and ministers see people at their best and their worst; that both are confided in and told things that people may not divulge to anyone else; and that both, at their best, are the recipients of much love and admiration from the public, in general, and from the individuals they work with, in particular. But they can also be the objects of great anger and scorn when the same public, patients, or parishioners believe their physicians or pastors have been negligent or motivated by money. My challenge was to find how to fulfill both callings and how much time to give to each.

For thirteen years, with much forbearance from family, friends, and colleagues, I was involved in both clinical practice and ministry. During that time, in 1988, Gloria and I were blessed with the opportunity to found a church in inner-city Boston. But the demands of ministry, not only to the church but to the surrounding community, became greater. As the strain of doing part-time medical ministry and full-time pastoral ministry increased, it became apparent that God was calling me to a different season in my life and that I had to make a choice. So, in 1992, at age forty-one, I gave up a successful and financially rewarding career as an emergency-room physician to become more fully the pastor of the Bethel African Methodist Episcopal Church. Was it a struggle? Yes, because I missed (and continue to miss) the people I worked with and the work to which I had given so many hours and from which I had learned so much. I must also admit some anxieties about my family's financial future. Was I sacrificing their future for the sake of my present pursuits? I thought, talked with others, and prayed long and hard about these and other questions. But having made the decision, I had few regrets. I would find out if I actually believed what I had been preaching all these years about trusting God, following Christ, and being empowered by the Spirit of God.

We call Bethel "a Bible-believing, Holy Spirit-empowered congregation." It is a family of three hundred members—adults and children from all walks of life, including the young and the elderly, high school dropouts and college and graduate students, married couples and single people, political refugees from several nations and young refugees from city streets. Most of the congregation is African American, but we also have white, Latino, and Asian members. We are a work in progress, a family in the making. Our challenge is to see if we can live up to our own statement of mission, which calls upon us to worship God, obey Christ, and serve others as we are led by the Holy Spirit. In the process we struggle to transcend the barriers of class, gender, and race at home while we build bridges of support to others as far away as Liberia, Ghana, Croatia, and the Philippines.

That commitment to transcending barriers is one of the reasons Bethel has so fully supported my involvement with the Ten Point Coalition as a founding officer and volunteer staff member. The coalition is a group of Christian clergy and laypeople from many denominations who are working together to help youth, and especially black youth, break free of urban violence and despair. The coalition was formed by twelve pastors from African American churches in Boston and Cambridge in response to two years of appalling violence. The breaking point came with a tragic incident at Morning Star Baptist Church in May 1992, when gang members disrupted a funeral and stabbed a rival gang member in the church. The reaction was anger and disbelief. A group of pastors, who had already been attempting for a year to connect with a generation of youth lost to the church, collaborated and produced a working paper that outlined ten programs that any congregation or organization can implement, singly or in combination. That plan included (1) adopting gangs; (2) commissioning missionaries to serve as advocates and mediators for black and Latino juveniles in the courts, working closely with probation officers; (3) commissioning youth workers to do street-level work with youth involved in drug trafficking; (4) establishing accountable, community-based economic development projects; (5) establishing partnerships among suburban, downtown, and inner-city churches as a means of providing spiritual, human, and material support; (6) initiating and supporting neighborhood crime-watch programs; (7) establishing working relationships between local churches and community-based health centers to provide pastoral counseling for families during time of crisis; (8) convening a working summit meeting for Christian black and Latino women and men to promote Christian sisterhoods and brotherhoods as rational alternatives to violent gang life; (9) establishing drop-in centers, services for battered women, and counseling for abusive men in churches; and (10) developing an aggressive black and Latino history curriculum to be taught in churches, with a focus on the struggles of women and poor people. These ten areas of work reflected what we had learned in more than a year of talking with gang leaders, drug dealers, their family members, the police, the courts, and the schools.

Over the past five years, the coalition has worked with congregations to implement all of the ten points. Church members and pastors have walked city streets; started summer and after-school programs that provide mentoring, tutoring, family support, job training, computer courses, math and science training, and music; mediated disputes between warring gangs; encouraged home ownership and local business development; become a presence in the courts; sponsored conferences on the church's response to domestic violence; started fatherhood training programs; and developed alternative sentencing programs. The success of these efforts has been integrally connected to the development of real partnerships with groups as diverse as the Archdiocese of Boston, the Jewish Community Relations Council, the Massachusetts Department of Probation, the Boston Rotary Club, Cooperative Metropolitan Ministries, the Boston Police Department, several universities, and a number of local and national businesses.

Boston's murder rate is now the lowest in thirty years, and violent crimes have dropped sharply, from 1,354 in 1990 to 516 in 1997. There were no juvenile gun homicides between 1995 and early 1998, though three were reported later that year. We are convinced that the work of the coalition has contributed to that dramatic reduction. And others seem to agree. In February 1997, Attorney General Janet Reno visited the Ten Point Coalition to see just how its many coordinated efforts had contributed to producing what many are calling the "Boston Miracle."

It is a miracle and a sign of what can happen when people of faith and commitment, from all walks of life, work together. It has been an opportunity for me to repay in part a great debt owed to those who purchased my life chances with shed blood and tears. It is also for me a reminder that the same God who afforded me the privilege of mending broken bodies has also given me the chance to mend broken spirits and prevent the breaking of bodies. I'm not sure why I have received these opportunities; I can only thank God that I have.

Gloria E. White-Hammond, M.D.

I am the third of eight children born to Wilbur and Mae White. My father was the son of Arkansas sharecroppers, my mother the daughter of Tennessee laborers. He was an air force sergeant; she was a homemaker. Dad's military career took us to various air bases—from Texas, where I was born; to Maine, where I started kindergarten; to Guam, the source of my fondest childhood memories; to New Hampshire, where we lived the longest; to Indiana, where I graduated from high school. I grew up feeling that there were many places to hang our hats, but no single location to call home. The entire world became our backyard.

I made the decision to become a doctor at the age of eight. Shy and insecure, I was usually the only black girl in my class, a combination that contributed to my sense of isolation. I remember lots of acquaintances but few friends. I was, however, an avid reader. Books were my tickets, and the library my vehicle, to a world of possibilities. One day, as a leggy, pigtailed grade-schooler, I picked out a blue book called *How to Become a Doctor*. The work sounded compelling, and the process of getting there seemed straightforward. Medicine would be my career of choice. My parents never discouraged me, even though none of us had ever seen a female or black physician. Collectively, we held fast to a dream that was fueled by faith.

Although I had been involved in Sunday school and youth groups all my life, I experienced my first "up close and personal" encounter with God when I was fifteen, just after my family had been transferred from New Hampshire to Indiana. The relocation proved extremely traumatic. In the middle of my sophomore year, I left behind a comfortable, established peer group in a New England seacoast city to face the unknown in a rural midwestern town. One evening, in the darkness of a dreary motel room, I found myself weeping desperately. I reached out to the television for companionship. Above the sound of my sobbing, I heard the evangelist Billy Graham offering a message of hope during an "Hour of Decision" crusade. I realized that this was *my* time to decide. I knelt down and asked God to remold my broken life and begin to lead me according to His will.

In 1968, I arrived at Boston University. In the wake of the assassination of Martin Luther King, I became one of the army of dream children that formed the largest class of black college students the nation had ever seen. It was an exhilarating but confusing season for this naive, timid young girl laboring to negotiate adolescence in the context of black power struggles and antiwar resistance. By the grace of God, I emerged from the experience with greater confidence. I felt proud to be black and privileged to be female. I was even more determined to capitalize on both of those strengths to become a physician in service, especially to other blacks.

That determination was reinforced during my junior year when I visited a newly developed, fledgling health center in Boston's South End. The center had been established by a grassroots organization with the help of a pediatrician and a retired businessman. These community activists had a vision for a facility that would provide high-quality, easily accessible, comprehensive health care for neighborhood residents. I called on the South End Community Health Center shortly after it opened and was privileged to meet Mel Scoville, the businessman, and Dr. Gerald Hass, the pediatrician. What I saw and heard during my brief visit came to be my benchmark as I continued to contemplate the kind of physician I would become and the nature and quality of my practice.

My junior year in college was monumental for yet another reason: that was the year I met the person who would become my most endearing friend. I was invited by a seminary student, Reverend John Bryant, to visit Saint Paul African Methodist Episcopal (A.M.E.) Church, where he was pastoring. He was eager for me to experience the fellowship there but also wanted to introduce me to a Harvard premedical student who was a member of the church. One spring evening, I elected to attend a concert being sponsored by the church. The choir was an all-male chorus from Morris Brown College in Atlanta. To be honest, I was less interested in the ministry and more interested in the men I hoped to meet, including the premed student I had heard about. That evening, Reverend Bryant introduced me to Ray Hammond, a tall, thin, pleasant young man who would be attending Harvard Medical School that fall. The guy was a real nerd. He was nice enough to befriend but decidedly not the type I would ever want to date. Over the next several months, however, I developed a wonderful relationship with Ray, who would eventually become not only my best friend but also my husband.

In 1972, I graduated from Boston University and matriculated at Tufts Medical School. Ray and I were married in 1973, at the end of his second year and my first year in medical school. Upon his graduation, he began his surgical residency at the New England Deaconess Hospital. A year later, I became a pediatric resident at the Boston Floating Hospital–New England Medical Center.

During those early years as a married couple, we began refining the art of juggling. Not only were we working at our residencies, but we were also active at Saint Paul, which by then had become our home church. Ray was on the ministerial staff; I was involved with the Missionary Society and ministry to new members. We were also resident tutors at one of the Harvard-Radcliffe dormitories, where we enjoyed a vibrant ministry to college students. At the end of my residency, I gave birth to our first daughter, Mariama. Mari was truly a gift from God.

I then spent the next two years at home being a full-time mom and continuing our work with the students. Ray and I became involved with a collaboration that subsequently became known as the Efficacy Institute. This group addressed issues of motivation and performance among students of color on both the college and high school levels.

The season for returning to medicine finally arrived. I promptly turned to the place that had made a space in my heart when the desire to become a doctor was much more dream than reality. Dr. Hass was still at the health center, which by that time had become known throughout the nation as a model for community medicine. In 1981 I joined the staff on a part-time basis and have continued there ever since. I remain firmly persuaded that the "chance" encounter at the

South End Community Health Center during my college years was actually designed to fertilize the seed first planted by that blue book. That seed would bear fruit years later when I returned to the clinic as a full-fledged physician.

In 1982, I gave birth to our second daughter, Adiya, another gift from God. That same year our lives took another twist when Ray was formally ordained as an itinerant elder in the A.M.E. Church. Shortly thereafter, he came to me with the proposition of starting a new church. He called it a vision—I called it a delusion. I had always imagined that he would practice medicine full-time while serving part-time as a ministerial assistant. Pastoring a start-up church required time-and-a-half, and several years elapsed before I caught the vision. Once I was on board, however, we moved forward to begin Bethel A.M.E. Church. The group of five that met in our dining room at our inaugural Bible study on June 16, 1988, has now grown to more than 250 wonderful congregants. What I initially perceived as my husband's foolishness has become a jewel in his crown of wisdom.

Bethel is a tremendous source of joy in my life and the life of our family. It comprises people who are determined to grow in their faith and are dedicated to putting that faith into action in their families and communities. Out of all of the contexts in which I have served —home, hospital, university, school—this is the one place where all the various strands have come together so beautifully. What so often seemed schizophrenic now feels visionary.

In April 1990, I went before our congregation to accept God's call to the ministry, to the surprise of few. It was simply a formal acknowledgment of what God had spoken into my heart several years earlier when, while still a resident, I saw God turn the saddest of natural circumstances into a tale of supernatural triumph.

During my residency, I met Elizabeth, a sensitive, pixielike five-year-old from Maine who had been diagnosed with a fatal form of leukemia. At best, our most potent chemotherapeutic protocols could buy her only a bit more time. During a hospitalization, Elizabeth and her mother awakened one morning with the same thought. They agreed to stop the chemotherapy and concentrate on enjoying the remaining time they had together as mother and daughter, friends, and confidantes. Reluctantly, the pediatric staff agreed to respect their decision.

Several months later I was making rounds on the oncology floor when I heard party sounds coming from one room. This was strange in a place where singing and laughter are not frequent visitors. I looked in to discover Elizabeth, in the midst of one last platelet infusion. She, her mother, and several friends and staff had donned party hats, as balloons floated overhead and cake was being distributed. Elizabeth invited me to join the fun and explained why they were having a party. While she had been praying (she paused to explain that praying means you talk to God and God talks back to you), God had told her she was going to go to heaven, where she would see her grandmother and would never be sick again. Although she had not been cured of the disease, Elizabeth had transcended the suffering to the place where celebration made sense. I was delighted to join the festivities.

Some time afterward, Elizabeth's mother paged me to the hospital lobby. I arrived to find her tenderly embracing a black Raggedy Ann doll. Elizabeth had died shortly after the party. Her mother explained that I was the first black person that Elizabeth had ever met. After we had become friends, Elizabeth bought this doll and named her Dr. Gloria. Before she died, Elizabeth made out a will, in which she willed Dr. Gloria to me. Dr. Gloria now sits in the big chair in my office. She reminds me of the defining moment when I realized that God had, indeed, marked out a path for me. The destination was not simply a career in medicine but a ministry of healing.

I have since spent my life seeking to fulfill that calling, particularly in addressing the needs of children. The South End Health Center is one of the venues where I work through that mission. For more than twenty-five years, the center has provided the highest-quality health care to those who have borne the brunt of the inadequacies of the American health-care system. For the past seventeen years I have striven to make my contribution to the cause. Most of my families are Latino and black. Sixty percent are on welfare. Thirty percent are among the working poor, with no medical insurance.

Most of my families do well. I marvel at their courage and tenacity to do so much with so little for so long. Too many of my families, however, do poorly. Five years ago, my inability to turn the tide in their lives precipitated a personal crisis. Too many of my children were succumbing to the risky behaviors that lead down the fast track to death and destruction at an early age. I was frustrated that my snapshot encounters, especially with bright, gifted teenage girls, seemed woefully inadequate. I felt baffled by the youth culture that would choose to say yes to drugs or promiscuity or school failure. Between the lines of our conversation I could hear their hurt and disappointment with themselves. It was not unlike the pain I had felt as an adolescent when I cried out to God from that lonely motel room. God had stepped in to address my grief during that crisis in my life. I asked him to use me to do likewise in the lives of other black adolescent girls.

This became the context for the formation of "Do the Write Thing," a creative-writing and mentoring ministry to adolescent girls considered to be at risk. For the past four years I have coordinated this intervention, which is sponsored by and meets at Bethel. At the outset, another member of our church and I mentored four young girls who were referred by the Boston Street Workers, a group assigned to help troubled young people and their families. This interaction has been marvelously rewarding, though extremely challenging. No sooner does a girl take three steps forward than she seems to take two steps back. Nevertheless, this push-and-pull has made the girls grow emotionally and spiritually. I am convinced that the key here is consistent, continuous, comprehensive ministry in the context of caring relationships. We now have five mentors working with twenty girls between the ages of thirteen and eighteen. Soon we shall begin working with young girls who are confined to residential juvenile detention centers.

So much more work has yet to be done—in my own life and the lives of our family, church, and community. But God has been amazingly gracious in bringing us this far by faith. The prospects for the journey ahead are extremely exciting. To God be the glory for the great things He has yet to do.

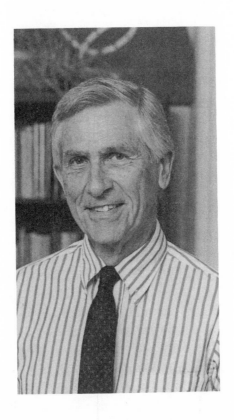

ALAN C. MERMANN became a chaplain at Yale University School of Medicine after a long career in pediatrics. He tells us of the people, events, and literary works that gradually focused his spiritual life and led to his dual career as a physician and minister. As a chaplain and pediatrician, Dr. Mermann is ideally suited to deal with the problems of medical students as they learn about life; he writes from a rich experience that explains how he can help heal the wounds of the medical training they must endure.

Looking for the Red Line

Alan C. Mermann, M.D.

> We never know how high we are
> Till we are asked to rise
> And then if we are true to plan
> Our statures touch the skies—
>
> —Emily Dickinson

In the days of sailing ships, when the Royal Navy ruled the seas, the best ropes, hawsers, and cables were identified by a red line running through them, signifying that they had been made for the navy and thereby assuring their integrity. This red line, a warrant for continuity and confidence, is a metaphor for the religious thread that I trace throughout my life. This life has been —and continues to be—rich and abundant with revelations about myself, my relationships, my work, and my faith.

As so often happens, an event, observation, or passing phrase crystallizes a vague collection of ideas into a pattern that makes sense for us. We hear a resonance, sense a cohesion, and we are enlightened. Certainly, artists can speak to this experience and to the anguish of waiting for it to occur. My recognition of the red line of faith in my life arrived late.

This particular experience of recognition came in spring 1979 as I wrote the personal statement that was to accompany my request to be ordained a minister of the United Church of Christ. The statement turned out to be a review of the journey I was on, one that began in my childhood and continued through my education, training, medical practice, marriage and family life, political and social concerns, and vocation to the ministry. It traced the development of my religious faith and outlined my reason for seeking ordination. Earlier, I had been challenged by the Committee on Church and Ministry when I sought in-care status, assuring my future ordainment: Why become a minister? Was it not possible to live a faithful life of loving service without the trappings of a minister? Jesus was a Galilean peasant and certainly not ordained in a Congregational church; why should I be? These questions, confronted in the ordination paper, revealed the red line in my life.

That line turned out to be a chain of persons, living and dead, who have been my teachers. In rereading the ordination paper, I was surprised to find no mention of my parents, whose influence on me, their only child, was considerable. Honest, intelligent, and working-class, they provided the physical and educational necessities of my life. In retrospect, however, their assistance in my emotional maturation was minimal, and they did little to encourage friendships with my peers. At that age I didn't know what I was missing; I spent my hours reading, walking the woods with my dog, and riding my bicycle. It was much later that I became aware of what I had lost out on during those years. My parents did not attend church and had no religious commitments. But as is still common practice, I was sent off to Sunday school in a nearby Presbyterian church, where I met my first teacher—and an enduring influence in my life.

Anna Ray Robinson, my Sunday school teacher and the wife of the minister, was a physician for the New York City Health Department as well as a Christian. I still have the Bible she gave to me as a Christmas gift in 1935. It is a lasting reminder of the start of my journey of faith. Over the years I have continued my study of newer translations of the Bible with increasingly sophisticated scholarship; I am not sure that my faith has matured to the same degree, although I live in hope.

The next person in this red line was another Sunday school teacher. Edwin Way Teale, a writer for *Popular Science,* taught the high school class at the Methodist Episcopal Church. His influence on us was extraordinary, and his stories of faith held us in amazed attention, revealing to us the meaning of faith in living our lives. Many of us returned to his classes during vacations from college. In 1946, my last year at Johns Hopkins School of Medicine, Mr. Teale gave me a copy of *Walden,* the American classic by Henry David Thoreau, as a Christmas gift. This book has been a scripture for me, instructing my understanding of self, world, and God.

I use the word *scripture* to classify *Walden* because, like the Bible, I examine *Walden* deeply. *Walden* is filled with metaphor; the book itself is a metaphor for the lived life. Thoreau must be read with great care: he means every word he writes. Words suggesting hesitancy or uncertainty—*could, might, some, possible, perhaps, awaken, morning, dawn, sleep*—contain the possibility for analogy, the fulcrum of a lever that could change a life. Thoreau wrote in earnest about the ease of wasting a life before its loftier goals are realized. Although he was not formally religious—he did not attend church—his sense of the spirit that infuses life, his devotion to all that lives, and his sensitivity to the created world have been instrumental in my journey of faith.

While living in Baltimore as a medical student, I attended the Mount Vernon Methodist Church. The senior pastor, Harold A. Bosley, was a leading light in his denomination and later became dean of Duke Divinity School. A thinker, a writer, and a superb preacher, he was available to me as I awakened to a world of poverty, suffering, and racial and religious prejudice and, simultaneously, to the discovery of my own loneliness and feelings of isolation. The red line was bringing me to a community of affection and support. My time with Bosley offered a foil that tested the meaning of faith amid the bad times. He showed me that the foundations of life must be sought, that one's personal scripture must be found and incorporated and that to know faith is possible. Thoreau teaches us to drive downward through the accepted foolishness, drivel, and inconsequential sideshows we believe to be real to find the bottom that will not fail. Like Jesus, who warns us to build our house not on sand, which washes away, but on a rock that will withstand the floods, Thoreau cautions us to make sure that we build our lives on a solid foundation.

Good preachers and Thoreau alike also warn us to awaken. Dawn, a recurring metaphor in *Walden,* is something we must awaken to if our lives are to be worthwhile. Only if we are awake can we be alive, alert to opportunity, available for learning, and present to those we serve. A necessary corollary to this is that we take control of our lives, continually evaluate who we are, and not be misled by appearances. We are called to be alert to interior questions—we must ask if the time has come for change. We must awake each day confident that our work and our life belong to us and that they are not impositions from outside the self.

Medical school was an obvious continuation of the red line of my life. The profound collegiality in the medical profession was exhilarating, as was living and working at Johns Hopkins, a school and hospital at the vanguard of contemporary American medical education and practice. At this point, a new figure worked his way into the red line.

At Hopkins, I was introduced to the writings of the Canadian physician William Osler, one of those responsible for Hopkins's renown. I frequently look at Sargent's painting *The Four Doctors* to recall the foundations of my training. At commencement we were given a copy of *Aequanimitas and Other Addresses*, a collection of Osler's essays. His delightful Victorian writings demand that we continue to study. Work, which he labeled the master word of medicine, is essential to being competent and learned in contemporary science and medicine. The image of Osler at McGill eating his lunch at the autopsy table is a charming reminder of the need for continuing study.

There were subtle spiritual components to Osler's life: a recognition of the passing away of all things, the choice of caring for the sick as a vocation, commitment to one's friends, and dedication to truth and knowledge—to the extent that they can be known. Osler's historical model was Sir Thomas Browne, the seventeenth-century English physician—perhaps also metaphysician—who wrote, among other works, the famous treatise *Religio Medici*. Possibly part of Osler's red line, Browne stressed the existence of two realities in which we live: "divided and distinguished worlds." Aware of the medieval Christian universe of magical faith, goblins, and mermaids, he also knew that the new science of the Enlightenment had arrived to change that world. I take Browne as a reliable example of one who holds two separate and distinct understandings of existence—physical and spiritual. He struggled to make sense of his life as a whole—the daily life of the physician accomplishing little and the life of faith lived in hope.

In 1954, in a lovely New England town, I opened a pediatric practice that in time expanded to five pediatricians. Along with my growing family, the practice occupied a large segment of my life. One day a week I worked in pediatric oncology at Yale–New Haven Hospital, where I had requested hospital privileges. I was fortunate to have as colleagues at Yale David Clement and Howard Pearson, both of whom were inspirational. Pediatric practice, particularly pediatric oncology, is sobering, encouraging, and humbling; I remain grateful to all the children and their parents whose suffering helped me grow —in learning and in spirit.

I was active in the Congregational church in our town, where I served as a deacon for a decade. I steadily read theology and social studies that reflected growing unrest in America. The bus boycott in Montgomery, integration in Little Rock, sit-ins in southern restaurants and drugstores, Freedom Riders, *Brown v. Board of Education* and, finally, Mississippi in the summer of 1964 opened my eyes to the crisis that was upon us. Deep within, I sensed that I was at a crossroads in my faith. If I ignored what was happening, I would remain outside the most significant societal event of my life. I made a decision: I chose to contribute slight skills and assistance to the ensuing struggles. As a member of the Medical Committee for Human Rights, I went to Alabama in 1966 to work with a Tuskegee Institute team studying the health and well-being of Lowndes County. The following year I joined a group of five other physicians examining the possibilities for preschool education for poor children. In the course of our study we discovered great hunger and deprivation. The testimony of our findings to a Senate subcommittee resulted in increased public assistance to the needy.

There were many other learning experiences packed into those years I worked in the South. My work there was yet another section in my red line. I was awestruck by the power of faith in the black persons I worked with; their churches struggled successfully to maintain a forgiving, hopeful attitude toward an aggressively hostile white population. I saw the emergence of a black power (quite different from the organized political group with the same name) that was developing political strength across the country. Eventually a door opened for me as I observed that religious faith could overcome terrible racial discrimination, that sacrifice was essential to the struggle for freedom, and that success would be known. In keeping with my education and my liberal political leanings, I had confidence that a government "of the people, by the people, and for the people" would solve these inequities. After all, hungry children are not easily ignored, or so I thought. Over time, when only small changes were being made and we began to give in gracefully to the status quo, I recalled the power I sensed in the small black churches I visited. I realized that the voices of black power were correct: the North had its own problems, many of which caused misery in the minority peoples we saw. I believed that nothing would happen unless our nation experienced a change of heart and mind; we would adjust to the pressure of the civil rights movement while the system remained in place. I searched for some way to bear witness to my faith amid the confusing times we were in, only to realize that I needed more religious education, particularly regarding my Christian heritage.

I applied for admission to Yale Divinity School in 1972 as a part-time student, since I was still practicing medicine. I started in the Master of Arts program, confident that I was there merely to learn about religion and its potential to bring change in our society. As fate would have it, my faculty adviser was a nun, Margaret Farley, one of America's leading ethicists. In our usually informal and infrequent conversations, she repeatedly posed the question: "Alan, why are you here?" As I contemplated the question, and my inadequate answers, I realized that something was going on in my life. I had heard the word *call* applied to ministers who said they were "called" to a church or to some other form of ministry. I understood that to be a euphemism for taking a job.

At the end of my first semester, however, I transferred to the Master of Divinity program. I had misunderstood the meaning of a calling and undervalued the power of realization. I did not expect to leave my medical practice: I was a physician and would always be. But now I felt the power of another demand. I decided to go in-care of the local association of Congregational ministers and see what happened. Then there was that question asked by a member of the committee: Why did I want to be a minister? Could I not serve my

God by my life as it was? I struggled with the question, finally realizing that I needed to be closer to the meaning of the life of Jesus in our world. It was as if I needed to move forward from the crowd around him, into a closer place where I could accept more responsibility for comprehending His mission. Perhaps I would know more of the pain and the feelings of inadequacy that are part of the experience. But I would have to do the work.

I was ordained in 1979 as assistant pastor in my local church. A special moment in the service served as a strong confirmation of my decision: the ordained ministers attending are invited to place their hands on the head of the newly ordained as a symbol of assurance and support. Surprised at the lightness of their touch, I recalled the laying on of hands forty years earlier when I first joined the church. I had an uncanny feeling of coming full circle from the first to the last promise of belief and hope for faith. The red line lengthened.

I continued to practice medicine, preached upon occasion, and sang in the choir. One day in my office, in the few moments between patients, I was looking out the window at a beautiful sugar maple in glowing fall colors. I was quite startled to hear myself saying aloud, "Is this it?" Apparently, a time for change was approaching, a new hour of decision.

A friend of mine who was leaving his position as chaplain of the Yale School of Medicine came by to see me one Sunday morning. While the school decided upon a new chaplain, he asked, would I be willing to keep his office open and running once a week? I agreed, and the inevitable occurred: I had the very clear, undeniable awareness that I was facing an opportunity for a ministry that was—literally —a calling. I took vacation time to think through what would be a major change in my life. While away, it became obvious that this was the calling that I had heard rumors of, had hoped for, and would accept. A significant part of making the decision was sharply focused prayer. I think we often speak of prayer with a certain embarrassment, an apologetic explanation of doing something that is not quite acceptable in our time of rational science and logical philosophy. But for those of us who have confidence in the existence of a knowable Creator and Sustainer who can be sensed in our interior self, prayer is an avenue for communication with assurance and expectation.

My discovery continues. The red line of my rope goes back to childhood: to teachers, to authors, to sacred texts, to promises, and to hopes. I have been graced with innumerable exemplars, teachers, witnesses, interrogators, pleaders, and presenters of gifts. All those known and unknown to me—that cloud of witnesses—contribute to my ongoing search for faith and courage. My work as chaplain at the medical school has been rewarding. Years of conversations with students continue to inform, awaken, and support me. The counseling that I do is sobering as I realize how talented and committed the students are. An unexpected coordinate appeared when I realized that my change of careers encouraged my students. When they applied to medical school, they assured their interviewers that they were committed to being physicians, whether clinicians or researchers. As a member of the admissions committee, I know the lingo well. But I am keenly aware of the diversity of talent and experience in these students' lives. Hearing them discuss the possibilities of several careers appeals to my sense of humor. One of the unexpected delights in my work as a Protestant minister is the opportunity for contact with Jewish students, particularly those of an Orthodox bent. They often find that the rabbi in their local synagogue tends to repeat the rules of the law when asked a difficult question about medical ethics, cadaver dissection, or other marginal religious issues. This offers little opportunity for debate; but to talk with a Christian opens all kinds of possibilities. Of course, it is the chaplain who learns the most from these encounters.

I live in hope that this thin red line of faith, this calling that goes back long before I knew it, will continue to sustain me. Perhaps we all need to look to the past to find the red line that tells us who we are and what we are to become. I am convinced that all of us have a calling to serve others, though hearing that call may be difficult. The source of our very being speaks to us in many and varied ways and eagerly awaits our decision to listen.

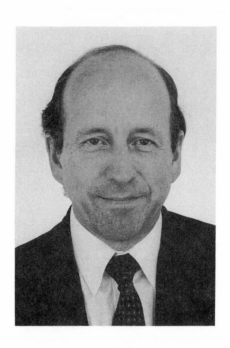

Each stage of his life, says JOHN L. YOUNG,

was built upon an earlier one. First came the religious

life, then priesthood in the Catholic Church; that was

followed by graduate education in science and finally

a medical degree from Stanford University. His

subsequent training in psychiatry led him to the field

of mental health. Currently he is an attending

psychiatrist at the Whiting Forensic Institute in

Middletown, Connecticut, an institution for the

criminally disturbed. Dr. Young has found fulfillment

in the combination of medicine and religion, both of

which occasionally foster remorse and encourage

goodness.

Priest in the Prison

John L. Young, M.D.

"You're surely working with the poorest of the poor," observed Peter A. Rosazza, auxiliary bishop of the Hartford Archdiocese, after ordaining a young member of my religious community, the Congregation of Holy Cross, to the priesthood. The statement startled me. Bishop Rosazza knew that I was assigned to work as a psychiatrist at the Whiting Forensic Institute in Middletown, Connecticut, the state's maximum-security hospital for the criminally insane. His words were confirming, however, because a priest's basic role is to extend and express the bishop's ministry. There he was, telling me that he recognized my medical work as a fulfillment of my mission as a priest. I would like more people to understand what this bishop saw so clearly. As a priest who went afield to express his priesthood through doctoring, I am eager to share my story—that of experiencing medical work as fundamentally religious or apostolic.

The care of psychiatric patients with legal problems, a growing subspecialty in forensic psychiatry, received formal recognition from the National Board of Medical Examiners in 1994. Although forensic psychiatry is ordinarily defined in terms of the use of psychiatric expertise to address legal questions for legal purposes, typically through consultation by an expert witness, it has traditionally included clinical practice in jails, prisons, and forensic hospitals. Fellowships in forensic psychiatry, for example, usually involve exposure to at least one of these settings.

The majority of patients I serve have been found not

guilty of serious criminal charges by reason of insanity. They have also been formally found dangerous enough to require confinement "for custody, care and treatment" in a maximum-security institution. Whiting Forensic Institute is a unique place to work. Passing through its metal detector and double gate soon becomes routine, and the ever-conscious need to preserve a safe environment becomes second nature. The twenty-five-year-old building holds one hundred beds for both male and female patients and is designed to appear and function as a mental health hospital rather than as a correction facility. There are no bars, and the facilities for sports, exercise, leather working, ceramics, arts and crafts, woodworking, and music are reasonably attractive; the patients' library, however, needs improvement. Overall, the effect is conducive to any of several modalities of treatment, all overseen by professional nurses, psychologists, social workers, and rehabilitation therapists.

Making a psychiatric contribution to this enterprise calls for a particular combination of skills and disposition. Every psychiatrist in the field would rank these skills differently. For me, the list begins with the ability to accept all comers — the situation is involuntary for the doctor as well as for the patient. Yet it is voluntary too: just as the doctor can choose to leave the whole situation for another job, the patient cannot be required to accept treatment. Although a criminal court chose to treat these individuals as patients by virtue of their mental illness, once in the hospital they are free to refuse all help, including medication. The forensic psychiatrist also has to be able to deal with, shall we say, less than deferential treatment by judges and opposing lawyers during hearings or courtroom appearances. This requires spiritual stamina, acquired through exposure and personal motivation.

More than in other inpatient settings, forensic patients tend to antagonize and endanger one another, a situation that calls for extra endurance and extraordinary patience on the part of everyone, qualities that must be not only instilled but sustained in the staff. I like to think of forensic hospital psychiatry as a process of reporting on a patient's behavior from the point of view of the entire treatment team, while providing strong support for the remediation of the patient's pathological behavior. In this role, the psychiatrist must wrestle with the conflicting roles of therapist and jailer and hone specialized skills. A healthy skepticism helps, as does the talent to interpret data on multiple levels and the ability to make judgments based on context as well as content.

Although this (or any) kind of work need not be an expression of one's personality, I find that it takes much of my personal talent and expresses the ultimate goals of my priesthood. For example, attending and presenting at professional conferences makes me a better priest as well as a more complete forensic psychiatrist. Similarly, clerical gatherings improve my work at the hospital. Although there is no single job that can fully represent the gospel, on my better days, forensic psychiatry offers me the opportunity to engage a large portion of it.

To be realistic, the gospel is not always discernible in my conduct. Like anyone else, I know that I can be difficult to get along with, and I am never eager for an assessment of my failings. On some days I feel empathic, enthusiastic, and helpful; on others I wish I had stayed at home. Not all my anger is righteous. I sometimes have to struggle to remain objective in the face of a patient's past savagery or, more difficult still, his or her current antics. In situations where stern communication is needed, however, I can often feel the urgency and power of God's kindness. Many times, the gospel has helped me successfully resolve a crisis. Meeting the personal and professional challenge of reflecting the gospel means becoming a better physician as well as a better priest.

To capture my life's work in a few words, I attempt to help human beings recognize one another's dignity and treat one another accordingly. The patients I treat are institutionalized because they have had major difficulty in this area. As a physician, I have the ability to treat the illness that put them there. As a priest, I want to conduct that treatment in a manner that reflects my religious values. It is my continued hope that I will grow as a forensic psychiatrist and a priest and, by pushing at the current frontiers, promote opportunity for others in my field to do likewise. The better the quality of my research, study, and caregiving, the more complete is the expression of my priesthood.

Offering Mass takes a few scant minutes; what happens the rest of the day should somehow be an extension of the saving sacrifice of

Christ's body and blood celebrated and remembered, offered and received. That does happen—however rarely and fleetingly—when one is working at one's best. I do not claim this experience only for myself or other clergy-physicians. Indeed, the church teaches that priesthood belongs to all believers.

People often ask whether my patients ever get better and leave the institution. My reply is that those who seriously want to generally can and do. Fortunately, those who refuse treatment are in the minority. To my surprise, it turned out that between 40 and 50 percent of the forty-odd patients who had come under my care in five years' time were approved for transfer from the maximum-security facility. As called for by the system, their next stop was a state hospital that had recently been upgraded to a medium-security level. Some of these patients have even been able to move back into the so-called community. A handful, however, have had to be returned to maximum security, half of them because of escape attempts and the other half because of transitional difficulties between settings. The disappointment of seeing this happen is only partly relieved by the conviction that it would be still worse to make the standards for recommending patient transfers too high.

I consider it important to study the outcome of my efforts, both the failures and the successes. This assessment occurs at several levels: as part of the day's work, through both structured and informal reflection, and even through that organized collegial enterprise called research. We have learned, for instance, that restricting the use of television leads to increased involvement in constructive therapeutic activities. With the help of colleagues, I have delved into such areas as injurious behavior patterns, parricide, pharmacologic treatment of aggression, and nonadherence to treatment.

People often ask about the tensions in being a priest and a physician. I do not feel any conflicts and have lately begun to speculate that their absence affirms my choice. Often I wish I had more time and energy to spend on untapped attractions. The opportunity to preach at Mass now comes about every few weeks and always leaves me feeling renewed and affirmed. Most days, on the way to or from work, I stop by church to pray; on days that I miss this personal moment, I feel frustration, but no anxiety.

When I was a seminarian, a spiritual director once told me, to my utter astonishment, that I ought to choose the ministry from which I could expect the most pleasure. That advice was a revelation: looking for satisfaction in my choice of vocation was legitimate. By way of further confirmation, much later I learned that the founder of our Holy Cross community, the Reverend Basil Moreau, had set up and directed a home for wayward boys outside Rome, at the special request of Pope Pius IX. The home had a vineyard called Vigna Pia, which provided what we would now call occupational therapy for the boys.

One of my classmates might be surprised to know how he taught me the value and joy of a good talk. Jesus, especially as portrayed in John's gospel with the likes of Nicodemus, the woman at the well, his mother, and his closest followers, obviously got involved in some very good talks. He also healed troubled minds along with ailing bodies, and I suspect that the physical healing followed from his spiritual action. Somehow, I am more aware of this when I pray than when I work, which must mean that the adage "to work is to pray" isn't completely true for me yet. There are nonetheless brief moments at work when it is true. As early as my rotation in obstetrics and gynecology, I found that presiding at childbirth was as intensely gripping as presiding at Mass. Similar moments of grace seem to occur during therapy. These remain quite distinct from the even more moving experiences I have ministering the Sacrament of Reconciliation.

It is also important to me that my work contribute to the ministry of my fellow clergy. For that to happen we must find ways to share our lives, which requires some effort. I hope that something of how I have learned to be present in my work comes across when we pray, socialize, and live together. As I write about my work and the issues it raises within religion and psychiatry, this group is part of my audience. At times, I can assist more directly; when I am called upon to function as a local superior, for example, my priestly responsibility involves gathering members for prayer and social time as well as supporting them in their apostolic works. Also, I help the body of the church by serving on the ethics committees of Catholic hospitals and by training and consulting with pastoral counselors.

Future alternatives and possibilities are exciting to contemplate.

Three or four books are urgently calling to be written, two of which have outlines. The topics range from New Haven's black clergy working in mental health ministries to inpatient care of dangerous psychiatric patients. I may expand my part-time teaching career. I could do much more as a consultant for public defenders on behalf of victims, as well as on behalf of mentally ill death-row inmates. I would enjoy helping impaired clergy, and I have lately wondered what it would be like to prepare and offer a religious retreat. If I continue working at the Whiting Institute, I shall be constantly challenged to keep up with psychiatry's accelerated growth as a scientific discipline. Whatever I do, I will want to increase my understanding of the spiritual possibilities in a marriage between psychiatry and religion.

Although I know no other individuals who have combined the priesthood and forensic psychiatry, I have always felt deeply comfortable with this synthesis. Each field brings much to the other: The awesome privilege of performing the sacrament of reconciliation ("hearing confessions") is enriched by the long hours spent trying to understand and help mend lives broken by mental illness severe enough to provoke legal problems. Fostering remorse and encouraging goodness are central aims for both priest and forensic mental health practitioner. Finding and encouraging the strengths of my patients builds my ability to help those in search of moral and spiritual growth. The psychological writings I discover consistently sustain my spirituality. In turn, spiritual reading relieves some of my hunger to learn more effective forensic psychiatry. Harvesting experiences from the two fields nourishes the discovery of fresh applications for both. They converge.

Part 6

Government and University

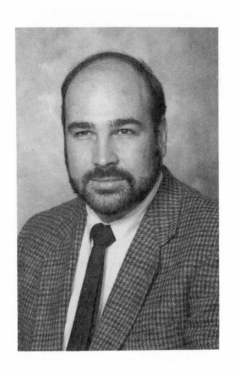

Although love of the outdoors made D A V I D   M .
A L B A L A consider a career in science and forestry, he
chose medicine in order to work directly with people.
After graduating from medical school, he spent time
in Nepal before training in urology. Currently Dr.
Albala is a urologist at Loyola University in Chicago.
In 1995–96 he became a White House Fellow and
special assistant to the secretary of transportation.
His experiences in drafting legislation, working on
health-related issues, and planning security for the
1996 Atlanta Olympic games have led him to a new
dream of a career in government.

Backpacking
to the Capital

David M. Albala, M.D.

I awoke to the sound of rain beating against my tent in the Smoky Mountains. More than a month had passed on my quest to hike the full 2,160 miles of the Appalachian Trail, from Springer Mountain, Georgia, to Baxter State Park, Maine. Resisting the temptation to go back to sleep, I went through the chores of making oatmeal in the rain, donning smelly hiking clothes, breaking camp, and stowing everything in my backpack before heading north once more. If there was a lesson to be gained from this long, hard trek, at age twenty-two, it was not yet apparent to me. When finally I stood atop Mount Katahdin, the northern terminus of the trail, my sense of accomplishment and joy was so strong that I can still feel it today. Only much later would I realize that the mental challenge and the sustained effort of those four and a half months had been the really hard parts and that persistence had been the key.

While hiking through parts of fourteen states, I was also struggling with the question of my future. At first, I thought of pursuing geology, my major in college, which would have allowed me to combine my strong interest in science with a love of the outdoors. My love of nature had led me, at eighteen, to work for the Appalachian Mountain Club, where I was in charge of a hostel visited by some ninety travelers daily. In dealing with diverse personalities, as well as feeding and educating large groups, I discovered an ability to organize and a desire to work with people.

In the following summers of my undergraduate years, my employer was the U.S. Forest Service in New Hampshire's White Mountains National Forest. Here, owing to my growing interest in working with people, my career choice gradually shifted toward forestry. Not that this was such a radical departure from my academic focus: both fields took a long-term view of the world, and both examined many of the same natural processes, from erosion to climatic changes to sudden cataclysms.

Finally, however, my two highest priorities of pursuing science and interacting with people converged, placing me on an altogether new path. One month before graduation from Lafayette University, I decided to study medicine.

Although my medical education took place at Brown University and, from my third year on, at Michigan State University in East Lansing, my most formative experience in becoming a doctor occurred during my senior year, through a program sponsored by Johns Hopkins. Under Dr. Jack Bryant, a pioneer of international medicine associated with the World Health Organization, I was part of a team that worked for two months to develop health-care programs in Nepal. In developing countries, where money is scarce, the ability to prioritize is paramount. In 1982 in Nepal, only about twelve cents per person was available for health care. By spending that money on the health of women and children, on immunization, and on the general level of hygiene, the impact was immediate. From there we expanded into basic health-care concerns for men and women.

Because most physicians and health-care workers in Nepal were in big cities like Katmandu, we developed programs and incentives to put doctors in rural areas, where they were desperately needed. We also trained community health workers to take care of routine needs, thereby freeing up physicians and nurses to go where they could do the most good.

My subsequent residency in urology at Dartmouth College was followed by a fellowship at Washington University in St. Louis. While I was at Dartmouth, Dr. Bryant reentered the picture by giving me an opportunity to return to Asia. This time the project involved a year in Pakistan and a new medical school, the Aga Khan University Medical Center in Karachi. There I not only taught students but also obtained funding for important projects. One grant underwrote the development of community-based health clinics in impoverished parts of Karachi and rural areas of Pakistan. Another grant was used to train Pakistani physicians in health-care development.

In 1991 I joined Loyola University in Chicago, where I have become an associate professor of urology. Loyola provided me with an opportunity to refine and expand my work with minimally invasive procedures. Another professional interest, and the one perhaps dearest to my heart, has been the screening program for prostate cancer in inner-city Chicago. Knowing how effective community-based clinics can be, we screen people at inner-city housing projects instead of expecting them to come to us. Gradually we gained acceptance in the community, and men once reluctant to go to a clinic began telling their friends about us. This screening program has grown steadily over the past seven years.

If any quality has seen me through life so far, it would have to be persistence. This also stood me in good stead when I applied to be a White House Fellow. Physicians all too often don't understand the workings of government, frequently perceiving it as a malign entity out to get them. Yet here was an opportunity to participate in shaping and implementing policy. Here was also a means to work with and for people on a much wider and thoroughly new plane.

I sent my first applications off with high hopes but was rejected several times. Finally, in autumn 1995, I found myself in Washington, D.C., one of fourteen Fellows. Recipients are assigned a one-year tenure in a department of government, where they may either work on a project that fits their training and experience or undertake a completely different program. I chose to work in the Department of Transportation (DOT) under Secretary Frederico Pena.

White House Fellows attend various meetings and social events that broaden their understanding of the workings of government. In my year, I met four presidents, the entire Supreme Court, General Colin Powell, and all members of the Cabinet, along with a host of prominent individuals such as Carl Sagan and Ralph Nader. Some speakers held controversial views, such as Dr. Jack Kevorkian or Dr. Henry Foster, nominated to be surgeon general but forced to withdraw because he had previously performed abortions. Dr. Foster had very telling remarks about the approval process that faces candidates for appointed office.

I found Secretary Pena to be a public servant in the truest sense, in that he very much cares about people. When transportation-related disasters occurred, he traveled to the site to be with those affected—for example, to Florida following the Value Jet crash and to Long Island after the TWA explosion.

In discussions of some DOT issues, my medical training provided a different point of view. For instance, most members of the National Transportation Safety Board are former pilots or engineers who utilize a certain methodology to learn what happens during a crash; I was able to provide some fresh insights from a medical perspective.

Another important project at the department involved automobile air bags, following the revelation that air bags may save adult lives but can kill young children who are not wearing seat belts in the front seat.

We also took up the question of whether the elderly should be allowed to drive if they have medical problems. The eye test required of all motorists, regardless of age, screens out the visually impaired. But what should be done about drivers with mild dementia caused by the aging process? Prohibiting the elderly from driving solely on the basis of age may limit their ability to function in society and may needlessly impinge upon their quality of life. Some drivers with mild to moderate impairment do adjust to their diminished skills, taking one particular route to the supermarket or doctor's office, or traveling only when traffic is light. After hearing expert opinions from around the country regarding the operation of airplanes, locomotives, and automobiles, we developed safety standards for operating a vehicle under certain medical conditions.

Workers sometimes contract an illness, usually respiratory in nature, from something in their workplace—a phenomenon known as "sick building syndrome." I treated one such building, none other than the headquarters of the DOT itself, which holds some fifteen hundred federal employees. After a number of workers fell ill, we traced the problem to a rare type of fungus in the walls near the gymnasium and devised a plan to eliminate the fungus.

Before the 1996 Olympic Games in Atlanta, we participated in an interagency review of security procedures. The sarin nerve-gas incident in the Tokyo subway had caused worldwide concern about possible chemical or biological terrorism. Planning ways to combat this threat involved visits to several locales in Atlanta.

At present, I hope to make some contribution to the ongoing national debate on health care, in which my understanding of the political system would inform my input as a physician. One of the biggest challenges will be developing a health-care system that provides universal coverage at a reasonable cost. The relationships of the various stakeholder groups will be important in the evolution of this system.

In Washington I worked with Senator William Frist (a Republican from Tennessee), a dynamic cardiac surgeon who believes in policy development as the best way to address health-care issues, an idea that also holds great appeal for me. A surgeon makes daily decisions that affect the lives of individual patients. On the other hand, a policy developer from the medical field could make decisions affecting lives on a national scale for a matter of years. He or she would need to combine an understanding of government operation with a commitment to helping people.

The diverse opportunities of my past have laid the unique foundations on which my medical career has been built. These opportunities have, I hope, made me a better physician. And what about taking on some further role in developing health-care policy on a federal level? This would be a subject well worth pondering over the course of a nice long hike.

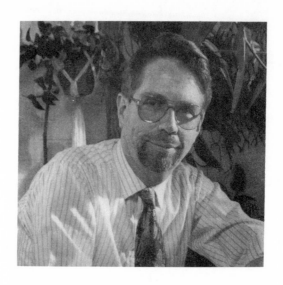

A physician-legislator in Arizona's House of Representatives, A N D R E W W . N I C H O L S is also involved
in public health, where the influence of the social order
on health and disease is most intense. With a medical
degree from Stanford and a master's degree in tropical
public health from Harvard, he is currently professor
of community medicine at the University of Arizona
College of Medicine. His strong interest in public
health led him to work toward the successful passage
of the Healthy Arizona Initiative in 1996. Selected as a
Henry Toll Fellow by the Council of State Governments
in 1996, Dr. Nichols has consistently worked for enact-
ment of progressive legislation in health, education, and
the environment. In November 1998 he was reelected
to his fourth term in the House of Representatives.

A Doctor in the House

Andrew W. Nichols, M.D.

believe that we all want to make a difference. This is why, in spite of initial discouragement and great personal expense, I fought for and won a seat in the Arizona state legislature. It is also why I entered the field of medicine in the first place and why I specialized in public health.

Early on, my family encouraged the idea of a career in community service. When I was a child, my Uncle Tom told me I had chosen well in wanting to practice the "second most noble profession" of medicine. The only higher calling, in his opinion, was the ministry, my maternal grandfather having set a good example as a minister in the Christian church. On the other hand, my paternal grandfather had long been a physician in my native town of Bardstown, Kentucky.

The question of pursuing medicine or the ministry was not settled until young adulthood. In high school my heroes were Harry Emerson Fosdick, the inspirational pastor of the Riverside Church in New York, and Albert Schweitzer, the medical missionary, theologian, philosopher, and musician, who energized a generation of followers. My closest boyhood friend once bought me a bust of the great humanitarian; this still holds a place of honor on my desk at home, along with many books detailing Dr. Schweitzer's philosophy.

During my college days, an invitation to visit the Union Theological Seminary in New York allowed me to meet my other hero, Dr. Fosdick, as well as the theologians Paul Tillich and Reinhold Niebuhr. One of my fondest memories is of the Sunday morning at Riverside Church when Dr. Fosdick, after the service, helped me put on my coat. What a thrill!

Medicine finally won out, with my acceptance in 1959 into the five-year medical curriculum at Stanford. Those were exciting days at the school. Professors included Joshua Lederberg and Arnold Kornberg, both of them Nobel Prize recipients; Don Kennedy, later the head of the Federal Drug Administration and president of Stanford University; and David Hamburg, who was to become president of the Carnegie Corporation of New York. I had role models in abundance.

The main influence on my future career direction, however, proved to be my work in preventive medicine in the developing world. Thanks to the International Tropical Medicine Program at Tulane University, during summer breaks at Stanford I traveled extensively, experiencing life in emerging nations. While sitting on a hillside in Guatemala, I determined that public health would be my career. Perhaps the frustration of seeing three or four people in a single bed at Roosevelt Hospital in Guatemala City had convinced me that conventional one-on-one therapy could not hope to address the magnitude of health problems around the globe. Also, I had reached an understanding of the connection between social order and health and of the inability of medical science per se to effect positive changes in that social order. And perhaps my theological side was coming out and calling me to a service beyond medicine, though one still rooted in the health field. Or did I believe that if I worked hard enough I could become a domestic Albert Schweitzer?

In any case, my decision to study public health was reinforced when, as an Eli Lilly Foundation Fellow, I spent a summer working at the Rio Verde Evangelical Hospital in Gois, Brazil. At Stanford I had seldom been in an operating room, but in Rio Verde, under the tutelage of Dr. Carlos Patricio, I was performing surgery, sometimes with an instruction book by my side, sometimes with instructions called out to me from the adjacent operatory. I realized then the difference between medicine in the field and medicine in the ivory tower, where interns and students had to await the privilege of assisting, however marginally, with a surgical procedure. According to Confucius, "I hear, I forget; I see, I remember; I do, I understand." In Brazil I gained new understanding of how doing leads to understanding and of how tenaciously missionary medicine had to labor to make a difference. Work in the field also made clear to me that many conditions whose cure lay only in surgery could be prevented in the first place through a healthy lifestyle, public education, and a clean environment, all of which could be promoted best through public health.

With public health as my long-term goal, I decided upon primary care as a good way to begin serving the underserved. I was accepted for a general medical internship at Saint Luke's Hospital in New York, which was closely affiliated with the Columbia University School of Physicians and Surgeons. Although Saint Luke's offered excellent training, internship and residency there were not easy. I became increasingly restive with what I saw as the irrelevancies of graduate medical education. I participated in rounds where attending faculty asked questions of house staff that could as easily have been answered by the patient, yet this was seldom done.

I took up the study of tropical medicine at Columbia's School of Public Health. Working under Dr. Harold "Stooly" Brown, professor of tropical medicine, I learned the importance of tropical diseases from a world perspective. Malaria, amebiasis, schistosomiasis, leishmaniasis, and a host of other diseases, extraordinarily widespread globally, were hardly touched upon in medical education in the United States. Fortunately, I had managed to combine a residency at Saint Luke's with a tropical medicine course at Columbia and public health training in New York City. This was to have a profound impact on my subsequent professional life.

Partway through my residency, I married, and my wife, Ann, and I enthusiastically joined the Peace Corps, in search of new vistas of shared experience and understanding. We were assigned to Peru. How memorable was that first trip to Cuzco! We flew in on a DC3 with no pressurization. The only oxygen came from tubes hanging from the ceiling. Suffering from high-altitude sickness, I—the Peace Corps doctor—was helped off the plane by an understanding bride and some bemused volunteers. The Peace Corps experience was under way.

In that first unforgettable year we traversed southwestern Peru, covering Lake Titicaca and the lakeside city of Puno, as well as the jungle cities of Tingo Maria and Puerto Maldonado. I learned to demand the right of way going up a mountain, because if you were pushed aside by a vehicle coming down, the drop could be several thousand feet. And I learned that if you accidentally ran your car into a human habitation or livestock compound, you drove away quickly if you valued your well-being.

In Peru I was the sole doctor to volunteers who often desperately needed medical care. During our second year, I became group leader for five U.S.-trained physicians serving around the country. While in Peru I treated my first cases of tapeworm and amebiasis. Diseases that had seemed so remote in medical school were now realities. Public health theory had become public health practice.

Ann and I also worked with the American Friends Service Committee in Peru, which afforded us valuable volunteer experience in the public health sector. I helped open a *barriada* (land invasion or slum) medical cooperative, and my wife helped establish a family planning program. The women in the barriada wanted to know why we had no children after a year of marriage. This was all the preamble Ann needed to captivate an audience. Although we were both totally exhausted and eager to see home again after two hard years in the Peace Corps, the experience was immensely satisfying.

In my last year at Saint Luke's, I was fortunate enough to meet a role model among physicians. Dr. Paul Torrens, director of the Community Medicine Program, shared all of my health-related interests. He was sensitive to the needs of the poor and conducted research on health-care issues; his program served people in the context of public health. Soon I was directing the first ambulatory Methadone Maintenance Program in New York and learning about the world of substance abuse. I also took a one-year public health residency at the New York City Health Department, where I rotated among various divisions, learning something from each. Dr. Torrens also encouraged me to coordinate a monthly seminar at Saint Luke's on issues affecting public health. Accordingly, some of New York's most renowned leaders in public health and social medicine shared their experience and perspective with our small group. This one-on-one contact did more than anything else to move me toward a career in academic community medicine and public health.

This also happened to be the year in which Mayor John Lindsey was voted out of office owing to the garbage strike, thus proving in the most visceral way that when environmental health issues are clearly grasped by the public, they transcend party affiliations and dominate the political process.

After Saint Luke's, a master's in public health seemed the next logical step. I entered the Harvard School of Public Health, where my most meaningful course was an elective in health-services administration. We designed our own curriculum and looked at new, planned communities such as Columbia, Maryland, and their health-care needs. Our aim was to create the best kind of health-care system, where all public health and service delivery functions were planned in advance and in partnership with the developing community. Our touchstone was early intervention through consultation.

The war on poverty was in full swing at this time, and the community health center movement had just begun. Dr. Herbert Adams, chair of the Department of Community Medicine at the University of Arizona College of Medicine, recruited me on the grounds that at age thirty-four I had had education enough: I should start applying my knowledge at his department's new community health center.

Service to the underserved became more of a priority for me than ever. I performed volunteer work at the El Rio Community Health Center in inner-city Tucson. The Christian Church, to which I belonged, had opened a nonprofit community clinic in the small town of Marana, thirty miles from Tucson, and I also volunteered there. Through association with the Arizona Migrant Ministry, donations of medicine arrived by the barrel from the Midwest, enabling the clinic to help the area's large itinerant population. My work in Marana rekindled the interest in rural health that had begun so many years earlier in Peru and Brazil.

My specialization in public health also gave me solutions to the problem of "publish or perish," since a young faculty member like me could not survive on teaching and service alone. Grants in health-services delivery research had not appealed to the rest of the faculty but were ideal for me. Also, I had the privilege of joining Drs. Hugh Smith and Lloyd Burton as a coauthor of the third edition of the textbook *Public Health and Community Medicine.* This project totally preoccupied me for several months as I learned the minuscule financial but tremendous intellectual rewards of authorship. I felt great pride and achievement on seeing my name on the cover of the published text.

Meanwhile, I found myself gravitating toward the public policy arena as my frustration increased at the insufficient money and support allotted to the causes dearest to me. Too many worthwhile health programs were being underfunded or going altogether unfunded by the state legislature. Equally apparent were the consequences of an inadequate public health infrastructure and the overfunding of highly specialized medical care delivery. These were the fundamental issues that led me to run for the Arizona state legislature.

On a more personal level, my single greatest inspiration to enter political life was Claire Dunn, a Catholic sister and teacher. Sister Claire had been elected to the legislature from my area, District 13, and had proven herself highly independent, hardworking, and effective. She had demonstrated a broad interest in the well-being of all the people in her district and the state. In 1981, she and another sister were instantly killed in a head-on collision on the freeway between Phoenix and Tucson. Hers was an example in public service that richly deserved to live on. (And, just perhaps, my decision to run had a genetic component. My father had been in the Kentucky state legislature and had once run for Congress.)

My first race, in 1982, was unsuccessful, though rewarding in some ways. In the course of visiting more than a thousand homes on countless evenings and weekends (often in 115-degree heat), I enjoyed spontaneous conversations on gun control, Arizona's abortion laws, and other "hot button" topics du jour. And certainly, nothing teaches humility better than a failed bid for office, especially after I had given it all I had, including ten thousand dollars of my own money and liberal contributions from friends and family.

In 1988 I ran again; my first try had been regarded as creditable, and by this time I had gained much more experience and backing. Hundreds of donors, coupled with a grassroots support group, made my prospects all the brighter, and, as before, I gave 100 percent of myself, as well as another ten thousand dollars of my own savings. I lost by approximately two hundred votes. This was a heartbreaker and should have spelled the end of my political career.

But if I can claim any quality in abundance, it must be persistence. At the risk of being dubbed the "Harold Stassen of Arizona Politics," I ran for a third time in 1992. At last, with the aid of the support group that had stuck with me since 1988, I led the ticket by a wide margin. When asked about the secret of my twice-deferred success, my answer was, "I fooled them into thinking that I was an incumbent. I ran so many times they didn't know the difference."

Now my doctor afield adventure had truly begun. A physician in the Arizona legislature was rare enough; there was only one other. A public health physician was unique. In my campaign I had stressed the need for a "Doctor in the House." In January 1993, upon being sworn in, I was assigned to the health and environmental committees. Subsequently, I was to receive appointments to the education and appropriation committees. Now I could accomplish much of what I had talked about, taught, and studied for so many years. No longer the supplicant before policy makers, I could influence those policies so consequential to the lives of my constituents.

Six years later, I can report substantial success. In terms of the environment, Arizona's solar energy leadership has been partially restored through a combination of tax incentives and policy directives. Further, both the air and water are cleaner than they were in 1992. I became a principal advocate for child health and safety, as well as expanded health coverage to the poor, with passage of a children's health insurance bill in 1998. And I have, suffice it to say, fought for "good" (and have helped defeat "bad") tobacco legislation. I have also consistently championed local versus state control of issues.

But in the field of health, Proposition 203, the Healthy Arizona Initiative, may stand as the strongest embodiment of my principles and aspirations. In addition to providing funding for six preventive health programs, the initiative offers medical coverage to a large number of Arizonans who are currently uninsured. The overwhelming passage of Proposition 203 by the people of Arizona in 1996 was predicated on the mobilization of a large and diverse constituency, including about forty health-related groups around the state. It also involved raising nearly a quarter of a million dollars to finance the initiative campaign. Later I was pleasantly surprised to learn that the project had won national visibility and has become a textbook example of successful community action for health at both the state and local levels.

Although I make every effort to keep my legislative and university duties separate, my professional concerns for public health cannot help but intersect with my legislative role. On winning a third term in the Arizona House of Representatives in 1996, I intensified my professionally based agenda for improved health and environmental conditions for the people of Arizona. Through lectures and site visits, I have also introduced students to the work of the legislature, thereby adding another dimension to my role as teacher. Advancing the cause of good public health, through the media forum provided by public office, has been emotionally and intellectually satisfying.

At this point, how do I feel about my work afield as a state legislator? Quite honestly, it continues to satisfy. Committee hearings bring an endless supply of information, as does contact with constituents and lobbyists. For those who are committed to learn, the legislature is a policy college.

Above all, the legislature offers an opportunity to make a difference. In countless ways, small efforts can reap big changes for a constituent or cause. And sometimes big efforts produce big results for the state and its people.

The fact that I continue to occupy a legislative office suggests that there is some advantage to being a "Doctor in the House," for my constituents and fellow legislators, as well as for myself. From my first days in the House, my colleagues have looked to me for answers regarding health-related issues. In general, we learn from one another; we serve one another.

I am often asked by other physicians, why run for office? There are more than enough good reasons. Run because an inner voice tells you to do so. Run because you must. Run to share your knowledge, but with a full awareness of the limits of that knowledge. Run in order to learn; it is the best adult-education program anywhere. Finally, run because you know that you can make a difference. What is more fulfilling than that?

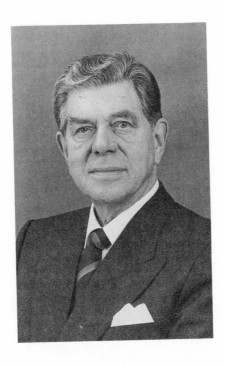

A virologist, university chancellor, and sculptor,

NILS OKER-BLOM (1919–95) spent almost his

entire career at the University of Helsinki. His daughter,

Teodora Oker-Blom, gives a loving account of his

many activities, from viral research at Yale University

and the Rockefeller Institute to his academic life in

Finland, where he was elected dean of the medical

school and then chancellor in 1983, the first physician

ever to hold this post. Oker-Blom devoted much of

his time to poetry, watercolors, and oil painting, along

with sculpture.

Nils Oker-Blom, M.D.

CARVING A NICHE,

IN CELLS AND BRONZE

Teodora Oker-Blom

I n summarizing the full and multifaceted life of my father, I have relied on published interviews and his own writings. Equally valuable were the discussions he and I had over the years, especially during summer holidays on our family island far out on the Finnish archipelago.

Nils, while still a child in Helsinki, was inspired to become a doctor by the example of the grandfather he had never met, Max Oker-Blom, who died two years before Nils was born. According to Nils's mother, Max was a physician who radiated empathy and "knew what people felt." His portrait stood watch in Nils's father's study and eventually in Nils's as well. My great-grandfather's many publications piqued my father's interest in medicine. Early on he read children's picture books about the structure and function of the human body; later, he turned to works by his grandfather, such as *Tales from a Doctor's Practice* and *The Medical Profession and Its Ethics*. Dedicated to social concerns as well as to science, Max was a pioneer in health and sex education. One of his more informal books, the title of which may be translated as *How My Family Doctor Told Me about Sexual Matters*, went through eighteen editions and was translated into ten languages.

Nils's other boyhood model was his great-grandfather, Christian Oker-Blom, a general of the infantry and the lord lieutenant of Viborg County. Christian also served as a senator in the late nineteenth century, when Finland was an autonomous grand duchy. Grandfather and great-grandfather instilled two major aspirations in Nils: to pursue a meaningful career and to serve his country.

His first years as a medical student at the University of Helsinki were interrupted by the Winter War in 1939. He went to the front as a junior doctor, attending to coastal artillery units. He subsequently resumed studies dealing with bacteriology, immune responses to bacterial infections, and antibody determinations for diagnostic purposes. Nils published his first papers on virology in 1949.

In 1949–50 Nils went to America to join the research laboratory of Francis Duran-Reynals at Yale. There he began to investigate the connection between viruses and cancer. In the words of Nils's student Ralf Pettersson (now head of the Ludwig Institute for Cancer Research in Stockholm), virology at this time was entering its golden age. When Nils returned to the University of Helsinki, he became involved with trials of the first antiviral medicines and of many effective vaccines and with developing efficient means of diagnosing viral infections. While chair of the university's Department of Virology (1957–83), he oversaw the descriptive cataloguing of the genetic structure of most pathogenic viruses.

Nils received various honors in recognition of his contributions to medicine and to numerous national and international organizations. In 1992 he was especially surprised and delighted when his medical colleagues voted him the Finnish title of *archiater*, an honor conferred on a ruler's personal physician in Egyptian, Greek, and Roman times. Only twelve doctors have held the office since it was first awarded in Finland in 1817. As archiater, Nils was able to address the public on the ethical and social concerns most important to him. He lectured throughout the country on the dangers of smoking and on the potential and thorny moral issues of gene technology and biotechnology.

In 1968, at age forty-nine, Nils was elected dean of the medical faculty at the University of Helsinki. In 1973 he became vice rector, and five years later rector, the first person chosen from the medical faculty in 140 years. His successor as chancellor, Lauri Saxen, described Nils as "impartial and just, conciliatory and constructive, gentlemanly and calm even amidst the most violent storms of academic controversy." It seems to me an appropriate description of the father I so admire.

As rector, Nils founded the university's Institute of Gene Technology in 1983. Here scientists from various faculties worked together, giving shape to his firm belief that a small country such as Finland could hold its own only through well-educated citizens and high-quality research facilities.

From 1983 to 1988, Nils was the first medical doctor to serve as chancellor of the university, its highest position. Among other duties, the chancellor represents the university at meetings of the national cabinet; the University of Helsinki is Finland's sole institution of higher learning to have a voice in the national government.

Nils felt strongly that education meant a well-rounded fostering of culture, transcending individual subjects. Its ultimate purpose was to produce citizens with an informed and critical view of their nation and the world. In this way Finland, as one of the more affluent nations, could act with moral responsibility in world affairs.

My father also expressed his lifelong love and support for the arts and humanities by founding the Athens Institute in Greece, which afforded Finnish and other international scholars a base for exploring classical Greek culture, thereby helping them gain a better perspective on their own heritage.

Art and literature always held a fascination for Nils. In younger days he had had his poetry published; one of his more emotive poems was set to music and for years was performed by a well-known Finnish singer.

His early days in medical practice led indirectly to one of his long-term creative passions. While serving as a temporary medical substitute in Finnish Lapland, Nils tried out the paints and brushes left behind by his predecessor. For decades he continued to paint, in both watercolor and oil. He was especially fond of the landscapes and seascapes around our summerhouse; he felt that his knowledge of anatomy gave him an advantage in life drawing.

This knowledge proved even more useful as painting gradually gave way to sculpture. Among my mother's relatives was a sculptor who, in the 1950s, influenced this change of artistic direction. Nils also learned much from the Finnish sculptor Wäinö Aaltonen, to whom he expressed his indebtedness in the essay "Why Do I Sculpt?" in the medical journal *Duodecim*.

The process of creativity in the arts and the sciences brought Nils similar trials and sorrows, and occasional triumphs. He sometimes quoted a verse by Aaltonen that graces the entrance to the Wäinö Aaltonen Museum in Turku:

Would that my heart were stone,
A rock cut with a vast and smiling face.
Time flows by. Alas, alas, if it were not so!
Its roots are wrenched by grief,
Yet it feels such hellish joy.

Here was the essence of the artist's quest for beauty, truth, and inner peace. Even if the struggle to create never brought completely satisfactory results, the work in itself was a source of joy and fulfillment. Nils professed this to be the case in his artistic as well as his scientific endeavors.

His sculptural efforts were rewarded by commissions from several departments at the University of Helsinki. The university also called on Nils to create half a dozen bronze medals to commemorate special occasions. The reproduction and sale of these medals (the proceeds of which he donated to the university) benefited the research projects of various campus foundations.

Reviewing a 1993 gallery exhibition of his work, the Finnish press wrote: "He is really a gifted sculptor and his bronzes and commemorative medals are very skillfully made. . . . One would not realize at once that this is work done by an amateur." Spurred on by this encouragement, he began two reliefs for the Athens Institute: one of the Finnish ambassador to Greece, who had been of great help to the institute, and one of himself. Unfortunately, Nils became ill and died in 1995, at age seventy-five, leaving these pieces unfinished. They were completed by his last teacher, Laila Pullinen, as a tribute to their friendship and were unveiled at the Athens Institute in March 1997.

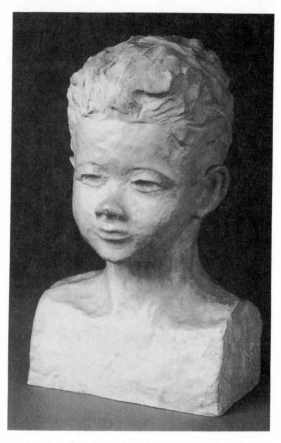

Nils Oker-Blom, sculpture of Max Oker-Blom,
the artist's son

My father put his heart and soul into everything he undertook and as a result was always in demand. He dreamed of a leisurely retirement in which he could concentrate on sculpting, but his professional and humanitarian concerns never gave him the opportunity. Even the honorary post of archiater entailed ongoing public duties. Family, friends, and colleagues marveled that pressure never seemed to faze him. Ever tactful, kind, and warm, my father exemplified the concept that life could indeed be an unqualified pleasure.

Part 7

Collecting

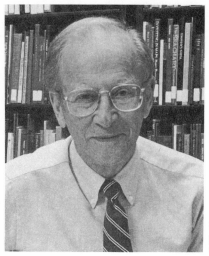

Libby Barrett

HAROLD L. OSHER was attracted to both medicine and maps as a child. After graduating from Boston University in 1947, he went on to specialize in cardiology. In his hometown of Portland, Maine, he continues to teach echocardiography part-time. In 1975, during a trip to London, he purchased his first antique map; over the years, his cartographic collection, one of the finest in the world, has grown to include maps, prints, and other historic documents. Wishing to preserve their remarkable acquisitions, he and his wife started the Osher Map Library at the University of Southern Maine, which contains some twenty thousand maps. Dr. Osher finds maps to be not only unique windows into history but remarkable works of art as well.

Afield with Old Maps

Harold L. Osher, M.D.

My interest in medicine was kindled during childhood by our family physician, a wise and gentle man whom I idolized. Early in my clinical training, cardiology became my focus; I was impressed with the power and precision of such diagnostic tools as cardiac catheterization and electrocardiography and with the availability of effective cardiac therapy. Here was a field at the vanguard of medical science. I could not have made a better choice; the endless breakthroughs and challenges of the past fifty years have been a continuing source of intellectual stimulation and satisfaction. I have seen our small community hospital evolve into a major university-affiliated tertiary medical center, where I eventually served as director of the cardiology division.

A parallel interest during my childhood was maps—road maps, National Geographic maps, and tourist maps gathered on trips. In the spring of 1975, while traveling in England, my wife and I visited the British Museum, where we encountered a wonderful exhibition of antique maps. On leaving the museum, still exhilarated by what we had seen, we happened upon a map and print shop. We ventured in and, at our request, were shown several old maps of our home state of Maine. As I scrutinized them, my wife encouraged me to buy them. Her words were: "If you like them so much, why don't you buy some?" And then, noting my hesitancy: "If you don't, I will!" Thus challenged, I boldly purchased two nineteenth-century maps of Maine for a total of twenty pounds sterling. We returned the following day and bought two eighteenth-century maps, a French map of New England and an English map of North America. I had no idea at the time that these would be anything more than isolated purchases.

Returning home, I bought several books on old maps, and the more I learned, the more fascinated I became with their enormous informational content and their importance as historical documents. My narrow geographic interest in Maine and New England progressively broadened to encompass the whole world, with emphasis on evolving geographic concepts. In time I was collecting the entire span of printed maps from the fifteenth through the twentieth centuries, especially those illustrating early exploration and discovery and those documenting other important historical events.

Eventually my wife and I realized that, without intending to do so, we had amassed a large and diversified collection, including a number of rare and important maps and atlases. We felt a sense of obligation to provide for appropriate long-term custody and use of these remarkable objects. We also wanted to preserve them where their historical value and their cultural and educational potential would be realized. Upon learning that the fine cartographic collection of Eleanor Houston and Lawrence M. C. Smith had been given to the University of Southern Maine (USM) in our hometown of Portland, we too donated our collection to the university and helped endow a facility to be known as the Osher Map Library and Smith Center for Cartographic Education. This facility, built in 1994 as part of a new library on the USM Portland campus, occupies approximately half the ground floor and contains a reference area, seminar room, staff offices, storage vault, preparation room for exhibits, and exhibition gallery, all in a secure, climate-controlled environment. The statement of purpose reads: "The Osher Map Library is committed to sharing its collection with a broad constituency by means of exhibitions, lectures, conferences, and other special events. . . . It serves the University community and residents of Maine and Northern New England, including the general public and local school systems, as well as the global community of scholars and researchers."

In accord with these goals, the library provides educational programs not only at the undergraduate and graduate college levels but also for primary and secondary schools. In addition, it is engaged in programs of scholarly research, publications, and free public exhibitions. My wife and I had the pleasure of curating the first three exhibitions, "Treasures of the Collection," "Maine 175," and "Jerusalem 3000" and of producing catalogs for the latter two. Dr. Matthew H. Edney, an internationally respected authority on geography and cartography, has been appointed faculty scholar in residence. He has developed an Internet web site containing information regarding the map library and its holdings, together with illustrated exhibition catalogs, and other educational materials. The library has thus extended into cyberspace.

The combined collections number approximately twenty thousand pre-1900 maps, either as separate sheets or as bound volumes. The latter include explorers' narratives, early travelers' accounts, and works on astronomy, geography, navigation, and history. The maps range in medium from a 1475 woodcut to modern satellite images. More than one hundred of the separate maps and more than fifty of the atlases and books date from before 1600; in addition, there are more than 100 terrestrial and celestial globes, along with a small collection of early surveying and navigational instruments. The collections provide a comprehensive basis for the study of Western cartography from its inception to modern times, beginning with early concepts of the world and focusing progressively on the New World, New England, and Maine.

My fascination with old maps is probably the consequence of a lifelong interest in history, together with a visual mind-set. It has always seemed to me that understanding historical events requires an appreciation of their temporal and spatial context. Maps are unique in that they provide such information in a graphic and comprehensible manner. They vividly portray regions varying in size from neighborhoods to the known universe, reflecting contemporary concepts as interpreted by mapmakers. Their informational content, however, goes far beyond geography, for they are often works of art that depict real or imaginary inhabitants and fauna and flora of distant lands; these works are sometimes further embellished with images of sailing ships, sea monsters, or allegorical figures from myth and legend. Maps were designed for many purposes: to illustrate and document evolving geographical concepts, discoveries, wars, conquests, and political events; to assert territorial claims, proclaim religious dogma, spread propaganda, promote colonization, or simply please the eye. They are extraordinarily rich sources of information about the world and its peoples over the centuries, encapsulating the ideology, culture, and scientific knowledge of the time. As such, they constitute unique portraits of past civilizations and therefore serve as powerful educational tools.

The multidimensional nature of maps is evident in "Nova Totius Terrarum Orbis Geographica AC Hydrographica," a hand-colored copperplate engraving from the seventeenth century, the golden age of Dutch cartography (plate 7). Engraved by Pieter van den Keere in 1608 and published in Amsterdam by Jan Jansson in 1630, it combines up-to-date geography with elegant design and skillful engraving. The many Latin inscriptions describe early explorations and discoveries and note geographical uncertainties. In addition to islands, the oceans are adorned with compass roses, masterful images of sailing ships, a South American native canoe, and a variety of sea monsters. The map itself is framed by a formal paneled border, a design known as *carte à figure*. Across the top, the "SEPTEM PLANETA" (seven planets—actually the five known planets plus the sun and the moon) are represented by mythological gods and goddesses. On the right side are allegorical representations of the four seasons, and on the left, personifications of the four classical elements of fire, air, water, and earth. Along the bottom are vignettes of the SEPTEM MIRABILIA MUNDI (the Seven Wonders of the Ancient World). This aesthetically pleasing map is replete with information from several disciplines, including geography, astronomy, anthropology, ancient and modern history, legend, and classical mythology. Careful scrutiny and study may be required to decode and interpret the graphics, in that images that appear to be purely decorative may in fact contain rich stores of information.

We are accustomed to seeing maps with north at the top. Ancient Arab and Chinese mapmakers, however, placed south at the top, and early European world maps were designed with east at the top, for several reasons. The sun rose in the east, and it was the supposed location of earthly paradise. In the case of maps of the Holy

Land, there was an additional reason: most pilgrims arrived on the Mediterranean coast at the port of Jaffa, so that their first view of the Holy Land was from the west, looking eastward. The words *orient* and *orientation* are derived from the Latin verb *oriri,* which means "to rise," referring to the sunrise in the East. In former times, one used a map with east at the top to orient oneself. This is exemplified by the oldest map in the library, one of a small number of surviving copies of the first modern printed map: "Cedar et tabernacla eius Aras wecha unde baldach in Job," a hand-colored woodcut that appeared in *Rudimentum Novitiorum,* a theological encyclopedia published in 1475 by Lucas Brandis in Lubeck, Germany (plate 8). The Holy Land is depicted in a bird's-eye view with east at the top and geographic landmarks represented as a mosaic of stylized hills. Jerusalem is portrayed as a circular walled city dominating the center of the map and overlooked by the Mount of Olives, with Bethlehem nearby on the right. Egypt and Gaza are in the lower right corner. At the port of Jaffa ("Japha," at the bottom center), pilgrims are disembarking from a galley. The walled city of Acre ("Accon") is to the left of Jerusalem, and Damascus is at the upper left border. Crudely illustrated biblical scenes include Egyptians drowning in the Red Sea (lower right); Moses receiving the Tablets of the Law on Mount Sinai, with God's face in the Burning Bush (upper right corner); spires of the submerged cities of Sodom and Gomorrah protruding from the Dead Sea (upper right); the Baptism of Jesus in the Jordan River (upper center); and the Crucifixion (below Jerusalem). Compass directions are indicated by eight personified "wind blowers" at the edges of the map, a convention replaced on later maps by compass roses.

Early maps were remarkably accurate, given the crude tools available to the surveyors, navigators, and mapmakers who produced them. Ancient civilizations were able to measure latitude by relatively simple astronomical observations, whereas longitudinal determinations required an accurate timepiece or chronometer, a device that was not invented until the latter part of the eighteenth century. Accordingly, early maps portrayed north-south relationships with reasonable accuracy, whereas estimates of east-west distances were largely guesswork. This deficiency was compounded by gaps in geographic knowledge, inaccurate observations, deliberately falsified reports, careless-ness, or wishful thinking. Some of the resulting maps depicted non-existent or mythical lands and waterways, such as Atlantis or a Northwest Passage connecting the Atlantic and Pacific Oceans across the top of North America. On other maps, real geographic features were omitted or distorted; for example, California was depicted as an island during much of the seventeenth century. Once introduced, er-rors were often perpetuated on later maps and had a significant im-pact on future exploration. Both the unexpected accuracy and the curious aberrations add to the fascination of early maps.

Some early maps exhibit what appear to be remarkable insights or prophetic depictions of yet undiscovered regions. For example, a sixteenth-century map showing a southern polar land mass closely resembling modern Antarctica is the result of an *inspired guess* by the great Flemish cartographer Gerard Mercator. Other sixteenth-century maps depict a "Strait of Anian" in the approximate position of the Bering Strait, which was not discovered until two centuries later; this is a coincidence resulting from an erroneous interpretation of Marco Polo's hearsay description of northeastern Asia. Another example is seen in a 1511 Spanish map of the Caribbean showing a land mass in the exact position of Florida. An accompanying note refers to the discovery of this land by a Spanish expedition at least two years before the 1513 visit of Juan Ponce de León in his search for the fountain of youth. This apparently precocious map is based on an overlooked historical event and thus represents the first docu-mentary evidence of the discovery of Florida.

In 1996 we had the good fortune to obtain a rare document known as the Columbus Letter. Published in Basel in 1494, it is a printed version of a letter written by Christopher Columbus in 1493, during his return voyage from the New World. A terrifying gale that blew up made him fear that his ship might sink and that the world would never learn of his great discoveries. He therefore wrote an ac-count of his voyage, placed it in a sealed cask, and threw it overboard, thinking that if his ship did indeed sink, there was at least a possi-bility that his exploits would become known. (The cask was never found.) Fortunately the storm abated, and after reaching port in

March 1493 Columbus sent a copy of his report in the form of a letter to King Ferdinand and Queen Isabella. The letter was made public, and printed versions were promptly issued in various European cities, generating great excitement. The editions published in Basel in 1493 and 1494 contained woodcut illustrations that are the first printed depictions of America and include a stylized pictorial map showing Columbus's ship among the islands of the West Indies— the first printed map of any part of the New World. This rare document is of special importance to students of American history, because it enables them to read Columbus's firsthand account of his historic voyage and to see, through his eyes, the first European view of the New World and its natives.

Physicians have for centuries played prominent roles in the history of cartography as mapmakers, publishers, scholars, and collectors. Among the more notable was Paolo Toscanelli (1397–1482), a Florentine physician, astronomer, and cosmographer who corresponded with Columbus and provided a map used in planning his historic voyage. In 1493 Dr. Hartmann Schedel (1449–1515) published the celebrated *Nuremberg Chronicle*, which contained among its more than eighteen hundred woodcuts an important early map of the known world. Michael Servetus (1511–53), a Spanish physician, theologian, and geographer, discovered pulmonary circulation and edited an influential textbook on geography. The personal library of Sir Hans Sloane (1660–1753), principal physician to King George II, contained a large map collection and became one of the foundations of the British Library. Dr. John Mitchell (1711–68), an American-born physician living in London, created the map that was used during negotiations of the boundaries of the newly independent United States; cartographic authorities have called this the most important map in American history. In a landmark of medical epidemiology, Dr. John Snow (1813–58) plotted the distribution of cholera cases on a map of London and thereby demonstrated their relationship to a contaminated water supply from the Broad Street pump; removal of the pump handle promptly terminated the cholera epidemic. The late Dr. Jonathan T. Lanman (1917–1988) was noted for his studies of portolan charts, the early coastal navigational documents produced in Europe, and for his book *Glimpses of History from Old Maps: A Collector's View;* his fine map and globe collection is now at his alma mater, Yale University.

In addition to my active role in the development and operation of the map library, I devote three days a week to medical practice. I therefore have the best of both worlds—involvement in my chosen field of medicine together with the excitement and intellectual stimulation of a new and rewarding endeavor. It may not be a coincidence that my medical and my afield activities have much in common; they are both graphically oriented combinations of art and science, and both involve teaching. I am grateful to my wife for encouraging me to develop an absorbing hobby in anticipation of the time when I would be partly or completely retired from my profession. I would otherwise have had a serious adjustment problem since I really had no active nonmedical intellectual interests before discovering maps.

A crucial factor in the success of our collecting has been the assistance we have received from map dealers. Not only have they encouraged, guided, and educated us, but, most important, they have located the increasingly scarce materials we were seeking. Although we have always derived pleasure from our collection, we came to regard ourselves as the privileged temporary custodians of objects that had a higher destiny. Consequently, it is a source of great satisfaction to us that the collection that we treasured so much will be preserved and will enrich the lives of generations of children and adults.

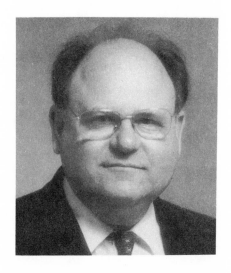

IRA REZAK, a professor of clinical medicine at the
State University of New York at Stony Brook, became
interested in coins during his youth in Brooklyn. The
chance acquisition of a Dutch guilder was to open a
world of discovery and self-determination. Whether
medals, tokens, badges, insignia, or a medium of
commerce, coins are part of history in that they
honor and memorialize prominent persons and
institutions. Dr. Rezak gives a comprehensive review
of the art and history of numismatics and tells how
collecting has enriched his understanding and practice
of medicine.

Mingling Medicine and Medals

Ira L. Rezak, M.D.

Some eccentric may find it wrong that a medical
doctor writes on a subject so remote from his profession but maybe he would not censure me so ar-
bitrarily if he considers that nobody is capable of
constant attention to such serious labor as is required in our profession. . . . Most who wrote
about medals were medical doctors, . . . [who]
have shown me the way.
—Charles Patin, *Introduction à l'histoire par la
connaissance des médailles* (Paris, 1665)

In an uncertain world, expertise and ownership often
support a sense of security and can determine status
and power. Deciding what we need to know and to
possess is a hallmark of our individuality. Such lessons
emerged in the course of my professional training as
a physician but also derive from my discovery in childhood of the pleasures of numismatics. This latter pursuit
has comforted, stimulated, and otherwise benefited me
for some fifty years. My numismatic career still vies for my
attention alongside my so-called principal profession,
medicine. There have been many interactions between the
two, and sometimes it's hard to tell which has the lead.

I was born in Brooklyn in 1938. As the eldest son of
a Jewish family recently arrived from Eastern Europe, I
felt that much was expected of me. I entered premedical
training perhaps less because of its ideals of science and

service and more because my immigrant father had hoped for achievement in that field himself. At that point, had I been left to my own devices, the humanities, teaching, or the law might have been likelier outcomes. In any case, I majored in history at Columbia University while pursuing my premed studies. Later, at the Albert Einstein College of Medicine, I settled on internal medicine. After a postinternship stint in the navy, I completed a medical residency, specializing in pulmonary diseases and, later, in critical care. In 1970, I joined the newly formed New York State Medical School at Stony Brook, Long Island, and its associated Veterans Administration Medical Center at Northport. My involvement in curricular planning, administration, and teaching, as well as the usual clinical tasks, made for a medical career as rich and satisfying as I could ever desire.

While still a schoolboy, I felt confined and burdened by my parents' insistence on self-discipline and hard work, but a means of liberation came to me, however inadvertently, via my grandfather. Each Hanukkah he gave me a silver dollar—an irresistible amount of spending power in those days of dime-a-week allowances. As a consequence, these coins were cashed in rather than hoarded year by year. When I was nine or ten, however, the bank stuck my grandfather with a Dutch 2 1/2 guilder, which looked like a dollar but, as I soon found out, couldn't be spent in Brooklyn. After frustration came curiosity about the strange language, coat of arms, and denomination that appeared on the unspendable coin. I went to the library by myself and, amazingly, was able to decode the coin; this led me to the revelation that I might know something important that my parents did not.

A world of my own, real but under my own control, had opened up to me: the world of collecting. Here was a piece of silver money, from thousands of miles away. I alone owned it, and the adults around me did not understand its significance. For many years thereafter, collecting coins proved to be just as rich in the thrills of discovery and possession, and intensely private. Secrecy was a key factor in escaping the control and authority of my parents. To them, such a hobby seemed a waste of time, a detriment to schoolwork, religious observance, and "proper play." Surreptitious collecting had an air of impropriety that was exciting. At the same time, numismatics proved to be an early expression of my individuality and self-determination. Gradually I grew less secretive and insular, at least among dealers, cognoscenti, and collecting peers. In return, I acquired new coins, useful information, and a burgeoning sense of confidence. I had been a shy child, but my progressive engagement with coins helped me enter the real world of social interactions, gratification, and occasional disappointment. I learned that I'd overpaid for some coins, and that foreign designs and exotic languages did not necessarily make a coin valuable. Increasing knowledge became an asset as I competed for bargains in shops and flea markets. I found myself gaining insight into budgeting, market fluctuations, and the ways of commerce.

I learned to be generous with information as I entered the more cooperative realm of premedical training. There the opportunity for friendly exchange became more valuable, and knowledge became more than a tool for gaining advantage. Eventually the self-esteem I gained through medical training, practice, and service helped me put my collecting in perspective: I began to view it as one of many possible intellectual and social explorations, not merely as an exercise in competitive possessiveness.

Coins are metal discs stamped exclusively by rulers (since about 600 B.C.) to assure people that the value of money is standardized and therefore trustworthy for commerce. Coins are the most available of numismatic objects and the type most often collected. It is hard to reckon precisely the number of coins ever made or extant today, but consider the coinage of the United States for a moment. It is among the more conservative in the modern world, changing little in design from year to year. Yet the United States in this century alone has produced about twenty-five regular coin types: three types of penny, three types of nickel, and so on up through now-obsolete silver and gold denominations. Such variety in coin issues escalates to twenty-five hundred if dates are taken into account, and up to more than five thousand if multiple mint marks and extraordinary commemorative coins are included. This crude extrapolation suggests the millions of coin varieties created since antiquity.

Availability is another matter. Great powers, from Periclean Athens and Rome through nineteenth-century Britain and twentieth-century America, may stamp millions of the same basic coin each year for decades, whereas obscure or transient polities leave few traces. After coins enter circulation, inadvertent losses, the subsequent melting of gold and silver coins, the systematic retirement of the coinage of defunct nations, and other factors affect the number of specimens that survive and thus the desirability, rarity, and cost of individual issues. Coins are not merely rare collectible artifacts, however. They depict and project persons and symbols, evoking in their past and present circulation social structures and aspirations. They are the earliest and most persistent form of reproduction, advertisement, and propaganda. Surviving pieces have actually participated in history.

It is striking that many of the founders of the science of numismatics were physicians. In the Renaissance, the acquisition of antiquities as objects of intellectual and aesthetic interest became a usual pursuit of gentlemen. Roman coins, commonly found in Italian soil, were the artifacts most widely and systematically acquired. The humanists who began this trend and the professionals and nobles who continued it included a high proportion of university graduates, among them physicians. These doctors, who were trained in language, history, and philosophy as well as the sciences, and who were accustomed to observing and categorizing, contributed much systematic scholarship to the literature of the humanities. *Médecins numismatistes* (1851) lists sixty-one physician-numismatists. Among them were Agricola, Arbuthnot, Bartholin, Hunter, Mead, and Rabelais. Perhaps the physicians' level of education, the requisite orderliness of their profession, their social status, and their access to leisure and money enabled them to be as sophisticated collectors of coins as they were of books and other scholarly paraphernalia.

Choosing what coins to collect is highly subjective, and the range of options is staggering. For me, collecting was initially an escape from Brooklyn. I was easily beguiled by the diversity, availability, and low cost of minor foreign coins. Later, larger, older, or special commemorative coins attracted me. Price became a greater factor too, for better coins, even in the good old days, were worth several dollars. I gradually became interested in other numismatic media, like medals, tokens, and badges. These, while metallic and coinlike, were not money per se. Since it is the history reflected in such objects that has been my abiding interest, and since all these nonmonetary items were less costly than rare coins, my collecting range broadened progressively.

Medals caught my attention around the time I entered medicine and for some forty years now have remained subjects of study for me. Unlike coins, medals are a medium of exchange and therefore need not be of small size, precious metal, or conservative design. Medals were originally bestowed as signs of personal favor by kings, emperors, and states and later by less regal persons and institutions. Gifts are ties that bind. But the medal has the unusual advantage of memorializing the importance of the donor: depicted on the medal is a person, sometimes represented symbolically. In preserving this durable, attractive object, the recipient is reminded of his or her relationship and obligation to the patron. The later collector of such an object holds in hand not only a piece of art but also a touchstone of past cultures, a record of the relationship between giver and recipient. The range of medallic art is wider than that of coins: portraiture; realistic and allegorical scenes; buildings; animal and vegetal themes; and a wide range of symbols.

One of my favorite medals is an award presented by the Royal Humane Society in 1788 to Mr. J. Young, a surgeon in London, for his successful resuscitation of Robert Miller, who had drowned in the Thames. Young used a variety of techniques promoted by the society, including warming the body, shaking the thorax, and sequential applications of "cordial confections and opening medicines," but his published report mentions that the patient's prompt response precluded any application of the society's "Medical Apparatus," an early form of mechanical ventilator. The Royal Humane Society, impressed by his "indefatigable professional application to every duty," awarded him its official Medal for Saving Life and appointed him medical assistant for districts between Westminster Bridge and Vauxhall. The image that appears on the medal, meant to be worn proudly by the awardee, is the apt emblem of the private "London Society for the Resuscitation of the Dying." It depicts a child carefully blowing on the waning ember of a torch in an attempt to bring it once again to full flame.

Specialization is almost inevitable in collecting today and, as in medicine, involves personal choice. I entered medicine as a generalist, though I later became a subspecialist in pulmonary disease and critical care, and have generally retained this original orientation. In numismatics, too, there is pride and reward in keeping a broad scope because of the quantity of materials to be examined and the opportunity to enhance one's collection and one's understanding of the material: the possibilities are limitless. But as with medicine, specialization has its advantages, in the form of more detailed expertise and a stronger sense of purpose or direction. In my own collecting I have remained a generalist but have given priority to objects and themes that reflect aspects of my heritage with which I particularly identify. These involve Russia, Judaism, and medicine. Russia represents an ancestral homeland, as well as a paradigm of that (admittedly idealized) exotic other that has long remained attractive to me as an alternative to the here and now. The Jewish community and religion have helped define me; certain pieces of my numismatic collection have afforded me a hands-on, in-depth engagement with Jewish material culture and history. Through a charity token in my collection, I have some connection with an eighteenth-century ghetto; with a prosperous sixteenth-century Jew of the Italian court; with whole communities in the dedication of new synagogues. By holding money virtually worn out by circulation within a Nazi concentration camp, I draw a bit closer to that experience. Numismatic tokens offer vicarious entries into my past and enhance an understanding of my present.

"Medicina in Nummis," medicine in numismatics, is the traditional term for the gathering of coins, medals, and other metallic artifacts of medical history. Ancient Greek and Roman cities were famous for their healing establishments: Pergamum, Kos, Epidaurus, Tiberias. They decorated their coinage with the caduceus of Aesculapius, the goddess Hygeia, their temples—all symbols of and advertisements for the effectiveness of their services. In other cultures, gods, saints, and their attributes have been displayed on coins, partly out of local pride but also because such images rendered the coins talismanic, possessed of healing virtues. They might protect the bearer from general harm or illness or might ward off a specific disease: Saint Roch for plague, Saint Anastasius for headache, Saint Vitus for epilepsy. In a ceremony promoted by the kings of England as late as the eighteenth century, gold coins depicting Saint Michael were the medium by which sufferers from tuberculous scrofula, known as "the king's evil," might be royally touched and healed. Tens of thousands of medals were also created to commemorate physicians, hospitals, almshouses, medical societies, and congresses. Many served generally as memorials, minimonuments, and souvenirs. Others were intended also to reward specific medical achievements, whether academic, clinical, or administrative. Upon their retirement from active practice or academic pursuits, prominent physicians from the late nineteenth century onward were often honored by their colleagues and former students at a large public banquet. As a souvenir of the event, a medal made especially for this dinner was presented in gold or silver to the honoree, and in bronze to the subscribers who attended. Such medals bear the person's portrait on one side and an indication of his or her accomplishments on the other. The medal of 1902 on the retirement of Dr. Jean Alfred Fournier (1832–1914), a senior practitioner at the Saint Louis Hospital in Paris and a specialist in venereal diseases, shows that solemnity was not the only commemorative mode available on such occasions. Fournier is realistically depicted in his office, and a discarded crutch indicates clinical success. While he wryly chides that he cannot completely defeat his adversary, Cupid nimbly scampers away, teasing the doctor with a blown kiss.

Numismatics may lead the physician-collector along wholly new avenues of understanding and experience. Comprehension of a primitive anticholera amulet of the last century requires anthropological as well as numismatic or medical knowledge. To hold a gold medal given to one of the few physicians who did not flee Memphis during the yellow fever epidemic of 1878 is to sense the role of courage in medical practice—a message that resonates in our own time.

The coin or medal records a historical moment in concrete form. Its interpretation is by no means necessarily straightforward. Consider a recent coin, a one-ounce South African gold Krugerrand depicting Paul Kruger, the Afrikaaner father of his country. In the future it may, as it does now, serve as an instrument of commerce. It may also remain a token of national prestige and wealth, or it may come to symbolize a vicious, oppressive, and defunct political system.

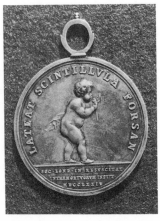 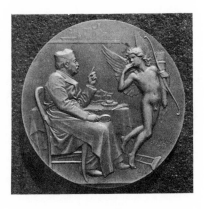

Silver medal by Lewis Pingo (left), created for the London Society for the
Resuscitation of Dying (The Royal Humane Society). The Latin
inscription reads: "Perhaps the little spark may be enhanced."

Bronze medal by Jules Clement Chaplain in honor of Jean Alfred
Fournier, syphilologist. Fournier is depicted chastizing Cupid,
who blows a kiss in return.

Such perspectives are all defensible and are not necessarily mutually
exclusive.

One hundred years ago, Warwick Wroth, a curator in the British
Museum, wrote that medals were "the mirrors which the men of the
past delighted to hold up to every momentous event, or to every
event which seemed to them momentous; and they are mirrors,
moreover, which have the magic power of still retaining the images
which they originally reflected." Today we have come to understand
that these medallic mirrors reflect all too well the reality they pur-
ported to describe, conveying the inevitable biases of those who
commissioned or used them. Medals—concrete, multiple, accessible
—are a particularly rich medium for discovering individual or societal self-perceptions, values, or biases.

When I was a child, collecting old things was considered to be
as valuable an activity as riding a hobby horse: it helped pass the time
but got you nowhere. Fifty years later, I know better. My career in
medicine has involved service to individual patients, students, colleagues, institutions, and society as a whole. There are great demands

and rewards, but the profession controls me rather than vice versa. My respite has been numismatics. I have chosen to invest energetically in this enterprise, studying, traveling, buying, and selling—in short, creating for myself a virtual profession. The rewards have been substantial, for in this microcosm I have encountered and contextualized art, history, commerce, and entire cultures, including my own. The methods of medicine and numismatics include order, precision, and the extrapolation that is their product. These techniques, applied within the humanistic context shared and valued by both disciplines, provide a means for enriching our lives and connecting us to something grander than ourselves.

Part 8

Fun and Games

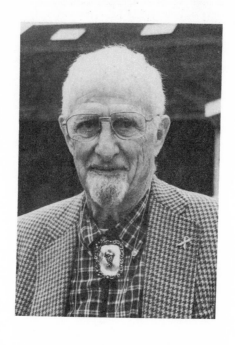

GEORGE W. NAUMBURG, JR., grew up on a farm in northern Westchester, New York. His banker father and his mother were both interested in psychoanalysis and, along with young George, underwent analysis. It was therefore natural for him to become a psychiatrist after graduating from the Yale School of Medicine. Yale also contributed to his career in wine making by providing him a background in chemistry and bacteriology. His Westchester vineyard is well known for its demanding standards and the continual improvement of the wines produced. As Naumburg notes, the wine maker learns very quickly, because the results can be tasted in a glass.

A Funny Thing Happened on the Way …

George W. Naumburg, Jr., M.D.

"When you can buy all the Château Mouton Rothschild you want for less money, why the hell do you want to start a vineyard?" my brother once asked. But wine making, or some similar pursuit afield, must have been in my blood, for I grew up on a farm. Home was Apple Bee Farm, in northern Westchester County, where I spent weekends and summers while attending school weekdays in Manhattan. The farm had cows, horses, chickens, pigs, apples, peaches, bees, a few grapes, vegetables, and my mother's beloved flower garden. In the days before balers, pitching hay onto the hay wagon, forkful by forkful, was the hardest work I had ever done, harder even than squeezing juice from grapes by hand.

Back in the roaring twenties we tried unsuccessfully to make beer; and our Concord grapes proved worthless for anything but jelly. Wine was available in my father's Prohibition-style wine cellar, with its secret door at the back of the coat closet. To be allowed into that sanctuary and bring up a bottle of scotch whiskey or French wine was a rite of passage. Prohibition was an exciting time. Our bootlegger was Grandfather Naumburg's coachman, and later his chauffeur. Prohibition brought him into a more lucrative business. My parents and Grandfather Morgenthau held that Prohibition was evil, worked to repeal it, and said that violating those laws whenever con-

217

venient was fine. Meanwhile Grandfather Naumburg was strictly law-abiding, although he would accept a bottle of Liebfraumilch from his sons. I found these contradictory views confusing.

At one point someone ran a still a mile upwind, hidden at the end of a dirt road. My father hated the stench of fermenting corn mash, so he called the Feds. Needing road directions, they arrived one morning in a big van to make the raid. Characteristically, the moonshiners had been warned; they had left hours before.

My father went to Exeter and Harvard, so that was where I went —no questions asked. Yale was my own choice for medical school. My father went into the family banking business on Wall Street but later grew interested in psychiatry and psychoanalysis. He wanted Exeter to add a psychiatrist to its medical staff, at his expense. The principal, Lewis Perry, repeatedly turned my father down, fearing that a psychiatrist would disrupt his efforts to build character in his students. Years later, my father did persuade him to have the school physician receive some training in child psychiatry. At the Hawthorne-Cedar Knolls School, then the Jewish Board of Guardians Home for Delinquents, he arranged, and paid for, the first staff psychiatrist in an institution for delinquents in America. He also financed early studies at Harvard aimed at identifying the determinants of delinquency. No doubt this sort of activity influenced my career choice.

At age fifteen I had another formative experience. I was taken to Mount Sinai Hospital with the bulbar form of poliomyelitis. In what was then the standard protocol, no one told me what was happening. Flowers came from Governor and Mrs. Herbert Lehman and from President and Mrs. Franklin Roosevelt, so I concluded I must have been pretty sick. The helplessness and isolation I experienced influenced my choice of medicine as a way to help others, by treating them better than I had been treated myself.

In the late 1960s I worked at Mount Sinai as liaison psychiatrist on the Adolescent Medical Unit. A number of adolescent patients were dying of acute lymphatic leukemia; as in my own case, no one discussed their condition with these patients. Because the nurses had to cope with a lot of depression, anger, misbehavior, and fear, I held weekly meetings to help deal with their feelings about the issues of death and dying. Often far from pleasant, these meetings were useful, for the nurses learned to cut through the adolescents' isolation and helplessness. The unit was located in the same building where I had survived my polio, at times making the meetings especially painful for me.

Another factor in my career choice arose soon after my arrival at Harvard: my parents divorced. I was well advised to seek help. During my Harvard years I went into Boston five times a week for psychoanalysis. This experience tipped the scale in favor of my going to medical school to specialize in psychiatry and psychoanalysis.

Harvard's school of medicine urged Harvard undergraduates to have an interview before making a formal application. The attitude of the interviewers, however, deterred me, and I never completed my application. At Yale I found the interviewers to be principally concerned with what the applicant, as a human being, had to offer the medical profession. One of my interviewers was a psychiatrist, and on hearing of my interest in the subject, he gave me some good advice: keep it to yourself. Psychiatrists were not yet welcomed into the medical profession.

On entering Yale's School of Medicine in the fall of 1941, I was informed that the students took no examinations. It dawned on me that I was now a responsible adult. The physiological chemistry and bacteriology I learned at Yale became as basic to my understanding of wine making as they were to my understanding of clinical medicine. Louis Pasteur's discoveries had been an important turning point for both disciplines; I entered medicine at another turning point. Sulfa drugs were in use, and antibiotics and corticosteroids were just arriving. Vineyards have increasingly effective herbicides and pesticides these days, but as yet nothing comparable to these medical innovations.

In my third year, I took a troubling issue to the department chair: Should my own emotional difficulties disqualify me from becoming a psychiatrist? He answered reassuringly, "How do you think the rest of us got here?"

Much later, considering my two children's medical education at the more traditional Mount Sinai, I realized that their years were a training, mine an education.

After Yale, assorted residencies, and a stint in the navy, I joined the new psychiatric unit at Mount Sinai Hospital, the first to be an integral part of a general hospital. The unit accepted any patient from within the hospital, no matter how disturbed or suicidal. A liaison psychiatrist was assigned to each ward unit as consultant. Psychosomatic medicine was in bloom, so we had our share of patients with ulcerative colitis and asthma.

A year later I started my psychoanalytic training at Columbia University. The length of time for training a psychoanalyst is matched only by the training of a Jesuit priest. For most students, an internship is followed by at least two years of psychiatric residence. At Columbia three half-day lectures each week continued for two years. My earlier psychoanalysis in Boston proved helpful, but this training required additional time on the couch. We also saw patients in a psychosomatic clinic and in psychotherapy, and each of us undertook the complete psychoanalysis of two patients. Theoretically, certification could be acquired in three years, but usually it took at least five. Although challenging, the process made us aware of ongoing improvement in our ability to diagnose and treat patients.

Eventually I shared an office with my friend and colleague Dick Frank. Mount Sinai had asked him to start an adolescent division, and he persuaded me to join him. We got the division functioning, and it provided good care and good training. Meanwhile, curious about what happened to patients in long-term institutional care, Dick and I set out to study individuals at the Linden Hill School in Westchester.

For the next fifteen years, my time was divided among this research, seeing my patients, and cultivating my wine. Finally, in 1988, at age seventy, I left the field of psychiatry. Even then, as my children said, I hadn't retired so much as reduced my workload to only one job.

By this time, my wife and I had started a vineyard and winery on a former dairy farm in North Salem, in northern Westchester County, not far from where I had grown up. Psychiatry during the week and grapes on weekends paralleled my childhood schedule: school in the city and weekends at the farm. In the spring of 1965 we planted six varieties of French hybrids that in three years would yield grapes for wine. Each spring we planted more vines, trying to farm what would grow well and produce acceptable wine in this untested area. We tried thirty-six varieties, including Chardonnay and other vinifera; the French hybrids proved to be best all around.

My knowledge of farming initiated a learning process that was furthered by reading, talking with people, attending meetings, and making mistakes. This new education included building trellises, training and pruning vines, diagnosing and treating diseases, and spraying, grafting, and protecting the vineyard from deer and birds. We are on a migratory flyway, which becomes especially active about three weeks before the grapes are ripe. One year, birds picked clean two acres of grapes in the course of one weekend. There was always something more to learn.

Within wine regions, wine growers share knowledge and facilities. In Westchester I have been quite isolated, though I can always count on Philip Wagner in Maryland and the New York State Agricultural Experiment Station in Geneva for help. I had not done lab work since my internship; now I was back at it in earnest. One produces better wines when acidity, pH, sugar content, and other variables are controlled. Each year brings the opportunity to correct the previous year's mistakes and deal with new problems.

In the vineyard cycle, pruning starts after Thanksgiving and continues until March. In May, ground temperature reaches fifty degrees and the vines start growing. From then through July, the vines are sprayed to keep the young leaves covered with fungicide. August is quiet, except for the installation of an electrical system to keep birds away. Late in August, the grapes are tested every few days for sugar content. Those for champagne are picked before the sugar gets too high. Cultivating the remaining grapes involves a balancing act between letting them ripen as long as possible and keeping rain, birds, or frost from damaging them. As of the second week in September, a dozen people are out picking.

The grapes go from the vineyard directly into a crusher-stemmer, after which they are seeded with a specific yeast and allowed to ferment for several days to pick up color and flavor from the skins. After pressing, the fermenting wine is stored in a closed stainless steel tank. The wine is inoculated with bacteria that metabolize the malic acid to lactic acid. After fermentation is complete, the wine must not come in contact with air, in that oxygen ruins wine and leaves, at best, some lovely vinegar. During the cold of winter, the doors of the winery are opened and the wine is chilled to cause precipitation of what you probably know as cream of tartar. Subsequently, the wine is filtered, blended, bottled, and labeled.

My farming experience had readied me for wine making but not for the attendant marketing. By 1979 we were selling grapes and juice to home wine makers and other wineries, and it seemed reasonable to assume that a satisfactory table wine from our vineyards would sell as well. Unfortunately, the mention of New York wine makes most people think of the sweet, kosher liquid made from Concord grapes. As a result, "pushing the product" has been a challenge. We have turned the former dairy barn into an attractive tasting room, where most of our wine is now sold. Visitors who sample our wine buy it and come back for more.

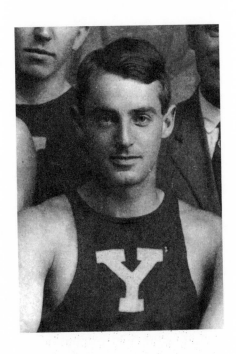

ALBERT C. GILBERT (1884–1961), better
known as "A.C.," graduated from Yale medical school
in 1909. He never practiced medicine, however, and
is far better known for his Erector Sets, chemistry sets,
and American Flyer electric trains. Jonathan Thomas
compiled the following essay from material provided
by Wm Brown, director of the Eli Whitney Museum,
who was kind enough to share details of Gilbert's
life. Brown finds a link between Gilbert's success as an
Olympian pole-vault champion and his career as a toy
maker. In manufacturing popular creative toys, Gilbert
liked to think that he gave millions of children a
healthy environment for learning.

A. C. Gilbert, M.D.

TYCOON OF TOYS

Jonathan A. Thomas

Alfred Carleton Gilbert was a man of diverse parts: showman, idealist, athlete, entrepreneur, and also a graduate of Yale Medical School. His avowed philosophy of life was, "Everything in life is a game, and the important thing is to win." Although he may no longer be a household name, he exerted a profound influence on the popular culture of the twentieth century. Several generations whose careers were shaped by childhood gifts of chemistry sets, Erector Sets, and his other educational toys stand in his debt. Yet this advocate of science and technology, of the "modern" world, was the product of a medical education unrecognizable as such by today's standards. Gilbert's medical background and training, however, were decisive in his life's work and gave credibility to his inventions and philosophy. He never practiced medicine, but his success owed much to the part of him that he could justifiably call physician.

According to his 1954 autobiography, *The Man Who Lives in Paradise*, Gilbert enjoyed a "frontier childhood" in Oregon. Such rustic chores as gathering firewood and bringing in the cows made him a robust youngster, though his father was a prosperous banker rather than a homesteader and could easily accommodate his son's interests and schooling. Gilbert's only "handicap" was his height of five feet seven inches, which he considered "modest" and which, he concedes, may have prompted him to compensate by trying to excel in other ways.

From early life, Gilbert strove to be the center of attention, and to this end he discovered two major outlets. A magic set, which was given to him as a prize for selling subscriptions to *Youth's Companion* magazine, revealed his knack for prestidigitation—a talent that served him well at college functions, on the vaudeville stage in New York and New Haven, and as an icebreaker at business meetings throughout his life. In a sense, magic was responsible for his medical degree: performing as a stage magician paid his way through Yale.

Gilbert also captured the spotlight through sports. At age twelve, he nearly ran away with a minstrel show as "Champion Boy Bag Puncher of the World." Talented in gymnastics, wrestling, football, and pole-vaulting, he set his share of world records and won a gold medal for pole-vaulting at the third modern Olympics in London in 1908, earning the congratulations of President Theodore Roosevelt. In a 1954 issue of the *New Yorker*, he went so far as to term himself a great pole-vaulting coach who also happened to run the world's largest toy company.

Sport was the all-important way station on Gilbert's road to medical school. In the nineteenth century, the fitness regimens of "Physical Culture" were widely regarded as a valid branch of health care. As systematized in Northern Europe, most notably by the German Ludwig Jahn, the seemingly ritualistic approach to dress, bathing, and movement bore some resemblance to yoga or tai chi, though it was grounded in contemporary science, as an attempt to remedy the pernicious effects of the Industrial Revolution on human health. Physical Culture's precept of "care for the body, settle the mind" foreshadowed both preventive and holistic medicine and offered a prescription for psychological well-being. And although Physical Culture attracted athletes like Gilbert, the recreational and competitive aspects of exercise were downplayed in favor of scientifically formulated healthy living.

The philosophy of Physical Culture figured in Gilbert's studio but was of less interest to him than the opportunity to learn from America's foremost wrestlers. All the same, he loved the forms of exercise that Physical Culture emphasized: chin-ups, bag punching, Indian clubs, and other means that allowed the ambitious young man to measure and compete against himself. And in light of Physical Culture's established place in the science of health, Gilbert was already pursuing studies that were largely equated in those days with at least one variety of medical training.

Gilbert began college at Pacific University, in Forest Grove, Oregon. In 1902 he attended a summer workshop at the Chautauqua Institute, in upstate New York. With roots in the nineteenth-century lyceum movement, Chautauqua had evolved into a center for various liberal and self-betterment programs. Blending serious and popular culture, the movement influenced people and ideas nationwide and continues to this day. Gilbert had chosen the center specifically for its School of Physical Education and the two-summer course it offers for training professional directors of physical education.

At Chautauqua, Gilbert met two representatives of Yale, Dr. W. G. Anderson and Dr. J. W. Seaver, director of the Yale Gymnasium. The three found common ground in their serious regard for sport, and Gilbert was enticed to enter Yale (technically, the Sheffield Scientific School affiliated with Yale) and study medicine. His long-term plan was to become a director of physical education, and to this end Seaver had convinced him that a medical degree was key if he wanted to become "the best possible director of physical education." Meanwhile, of course, he would play football and other sports for Yale.

Today the training of doctors and physical instructors seems altogether unconnected, but under the influence of Physical Culture, physical education was an accepted medical specialization and would remain so until the rejection of all things German in World War I. As of 1905, when Gilbert entered Yale, aspirin and the sphygmomanometer were the latest innovations. It was still the age of Pasteur, Lister, and Röntgen. Just outside the bounds of conventional medicine flourished "wellness" cults like that of the eccentric Will Keith Kellogg, who prescribed abstinence, electric shocks, and whole-grain cereals. Wellness, of course, has had a renaissance in the last part of the twentieth century as well.

Perhaps it was the unsophisticated state of medical science that prompted Gilbert, after receiving his M.D. in 1909, to regard it as no more important than various other career paths, no better than any number of alternatives for being of use in the world. Nonetheless, at Yale, Gilbert applied himself to the fullest. He not only established himself a champion at wrestling, gymnastics, Indian clubs, and pole-vaulting (at the Olympic level) but also excelled in chemistry, biology, and physics courses, graduating with high honors. His thesis, *The Genito-Urinary Phenomena of Athletes: Associated Symptoms, Sequel and Significance,* reflected his era's close links between athletics and medical practice. His yearbook states that he "was voted as having done the most for Yale of his class."

Still, his autobiography makes little of his medical studies, mentioning that he might have excelled at surgery and that medicine had distracted him from going further in football. As for his avowed plan of going into physical education, his restless, ambitious spirit seemed more inclined to seize on promising opportunities as they came to hand. His first endeavor, immediately after graduation, was to help form the Mysto Magic Company (in Westville, Connecticut), which produced materials for stage and amateur magicians. This was the forerunner of his immensely successful A. C. Gilbert Manufacturing Company in New Haven.

Although his subsequent business ventures were marked by finely calculated self-promotion, turning him into a national celebrity, Gilbert was also imbued with a concern for both individual and social welfare, arguably an extension of the compassion and idealism cultivated during his medical training. Even as Henry Ford created vehicles for everyone, Gilbert democratized the use of toys, though they still remained relatively expensive at a time of improved purchasing power. He argued for the educational role of toys in preparing future builders and leaders. Inspired by the towering steel construction under way in New York, he invented the Erector Set, thereby putting electric motors in the hands of boys whose fathers had known only the power of water or steam. In 1920s society, this was progressive thinking, comparable to giving computers to school-children today.

Dozens of other affordable, instructional toys followed, includ-

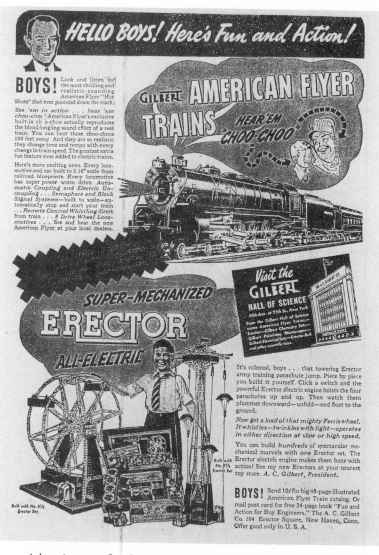

Advertisement for the Erector Set and American Flyer trains,
creations of A. C. Gilbert.

ing chemistry sets and American Flyer trains. "Learn to master this
toy, and you will be master of your life," Gilbert proclaimed in his
products' instruction manuals. Tied in with this message, he also
praised the rewards of hard work, fitness, and healthy living in his
radio interviews and magazine advertisements. Through his "Gilbert

Institute of Toy Engineering," degrees, diplomas, and prizes went to children who had reached certain stages of mastery in the use of his educational toys.

To Gilbert, healthy play was intimately linked with the well-being of mind and body, an extension of the principle of "care for the body, settle the mind." Like sports, play could benefit not only the individual but also society, by firing the imaginations of children and guiding them along paths to meaningful vocations, to innovation and invention.

A brilliant aspect of Gilbert's appeal was his use of the kindly, authoritative tone of the family physician. More than gimmickry was involved here, however. Motivations of fame and profit were inextricably mingled with a genuine concern for society. In his public endorsements of physical exercise, and in his belief that an everyday activity such as play contributed to individual well-being as well as to the long-term betterment of society, Gilbert was proceeding from his philosophy of medicine learned early at Chautauqua and Yale. They served him well for the next fifty years.

Contributors

DAVID M. ALBALA, M.D., associate professor of urology, Loyola University Medical Center, Maywood, Illinois

ANDREA M. BALDECK, M.D., anesthesiologist (retired); photographer, Blue Bell, Pennsylvania

ELAINE L. BEARER, M.D., PH.D., Department of Pathology and Laboratory Medicine, Brown University, Providence, Rhode Island

WM BROWN, director, Eli Whitney Museum, Hamden, Connecticut

SIR ROY CALNE, M.D., Department of Surgery, Douglas House Annex, Cambridge, England

RAFAEL CAMPO, M.D., Division of General Internal Medicine, Beth Israel Deaconess Medical Center Hospital, Boston, Massachusetts

JAMES J. CERDA, M.D., gastroenterologist, professor of medicine, University of Florida College of Medicine, Gainesville, Florida

ERNEST CRAIGE, M.D., professor of medicine emeritus (cardiology), University of North Carolina School of Medicine, Chapel Hill, North Carolina

MARY G. MCCREA CURNEN, M.D., DR.P.H., clinical professor of epidemiology and pediatrics, associate director of the Program for Humanities in Medicine at Yale University School of Medicine, New Haven, Connecticut

THOMAS P. DUFFY, M.D., professor of internal medicine (hematology) and medical director of the Program for Humanities in Medicine at Yale University School of Medicine, New Haven, Connecticut

THE REVEREND RAY A. HAMMOND, M.A., M.D., emergency physician (retired); pastor, Bethel African Methodist Episcopal Church, Boston, Massachusetts

MICHAEL A. LACOMBE, M.D., general internist, writer, Bridgton, Maine

ALICE LEVINE, M.D., endocrinologist, associate professor of medicine, Mount Sinai School of Medicine, New York, New York

SHEILA LENNON, M.ED., teacher, writer, Providence, Rhode Island

HARVEY MANDELL, M.D., internist (retired), Norwich, Connecticut

THE REVEREND ALAN C. MERMANN, M.D., S.T.M., M. DIV., chaplain, Yale University School of Medicine; pediatrician (retired), New Haven, Connecticut

GEORGE W. NAUMBURG, JR., M.D., associate clinical professor, adolescent psychiatry, Mount Sinai School of Medicine (retired); wine maker, North Salem, New York

ELI NEWBERGER, M.D., pediatrician; director, Family Development Program, Children's Hospital, Boston, Massachusetts

ANDREW W. NICHOLS, M.D., M.P.H., public health physician; professor and director, Rural Health Office, College of Medicine, University of Arizona Health Sciences Center, Tucson, Arizona; representative, House of Representatives, Arizona State Legislature

TEODORA OKER-BLOM, director, Karolinska Institute Library and Information Center, Sweden

HAROLD L. OSHER, M.D., director (emeritus) of cardiology, Maine Medical Center; founder, Osher Map Library, University of Southern Maine, Portland, Maine

IRA L. REZAK, M.D., professor of clinical medicine (pulmonary disease), School of Medicine, State University of New York at Stony Brook, New York

DEBORAH ST. JAMES, B.A., writer, editor, and educator; manager, Continuing Education at Bayer Pharmaceutical, Inc., West Haven, Connecticut

WAYNE O. SOUTHWICK, M.D., professor emeritus of orthopedic surgery, Yale University School of Medicine, New Haven, Connecticut

HOWARD SPIRO, M.D., professor of medicine, director of the Program for Humanities in Medicine at Yale University School of Medicine, New Haven, Connecticut

MARK H. SWARTZ, M.D., professor of medicine (cardiology), Morchand professor of medical education, and director, The Morchand Center for Clinical Competence; dean for Continuing Medical Education, Mount Sinai School of Medicine, New York, New York

JONATHAN A. THOMAS, M.A., freelance writer and copyeditor, Providence, Rhode Island

WILLIAM THORNTON, M.D., NASA scientist-astronaut (retired); clinical professor of medicine, University of Texas Medical Branch, Galveston, Texas

F. NORMAN VICKERS, M.D., gastroenterologist, Pensacola, Florida

GERALD WEISSMANN, M.D., professor of medicine, director, Division of Rheumatology, Department of Medicine, New York University Medical Center, New York; trustee, Marine Biological Laboratory, Woods Hole, Massachusetts

THE REVEREND GLORIA E. WHITE-HAMMOND, M.D., M.DIV., pastor, Bethel African Methodist Episcopal Church; pediatrician, South End Health Center, Boston, Massachusetts

BARBARA YOUNG, M.D., psychiatrist and psychoanalyst (semi-retired); assistant professor in psychiatry, Johns Hopkins School of Medicine; photographer, Baltimore, Maryland

THE REVEREND JOHN L. YOUNG, M.D., attending psychiatrist, Whiting Forensic Division of Connecticut Valley Hospital; priest, Middletown, Connecticut